The 10-Day Green Smoothie Cleanse For Weight Loss

10 Day Diet Plan+50 Delicious Quick & Easy Smoothie Recipes For Weight Loss

Table of Contents

Chapter 4: Detox Green Smoothies Recipes For Weight Loss 82

Introduction

This diet plan, as evident from its name, is based on water, fruits, and green leafy veggies. The main goal of the 10-Day Green Smoothie Cleanse Weight Loss Diet Plan is to cleanse and detox your body to help you lose weight and improve your overall health.

Chapter 1: About The 10-day Green Smoothie Cleanse Weight Loss Diet Plan

The 10-Day Green Smoothie Cleanse Weight Loss Diet Plan can be followed in two different ways. The first plan consists of only leafy green smoothies and a light snack per day while the modified plan consists of smoothies, snacks, and one healthy meal a day. To properly follow this diet, you need to eliminate processed foods and add natural produce and healthy fats to your daily diet while keeping your sugar intake low. This will make your weight loss easier.

What laid the foundation of the 10-day Green smoothie Cleanse Weight loss Diet Plan?

In order to properly lose weight, your body has to detoxify itself first. . This means that your body needs to purge itself of toxins that have built up over time from unhealthy habits and diets.

It is very hard to remove toxins from the fat stored in cells by only changing your diet plan so you have to detox it first. Raw green veggies are known to be beneficial for this process as well as for introducing vital nutrients into your body. More so, eliminating certain foods from your diet for a period of ten days can push you closer to your goal. At the same time, your taste buds will get reprogrammed to enjoy and crave nutrient-rich healthy foods over processed unhealthy options.

This program is made so you don't have to worry about counting calories or adopting unsustainable lifetime diet plans. In fact, you'll likely find yourself choosing healthier foods on your own after your 10-

day cleanse as your body will be so used to the nutrients that it will no longer be satisfied by other foods.

The 10-Day Green Smoothie Cleanse Weight Loss Diet Plan Options

There are two different options for this 10-day cleanse that you can choose between based on how strong you want your cleanse to be. There are also different food restrictions and allowances for each option that you should consider, too. The two options are the Full Cleanse Plan and the Modified Cleanse Plan.

- **Full Cleanse Plan:**
In this diet plan, you are only allowed to have smoothies, tea or water, and certain snacks for the full 10 days.

- **Modified Cleanse:**
In this diet plan, you are allowed to have two smoothies for both breakfast and lunch, one healthy natural-food meal for dinner, tea or water, and certain snacks for the full 10 days. As you can see, this one is a little more lenient.

Foods to Eat and Foods Not to Eat on the Full Cleanse Plan

In the full cleanse variant of the plan, your daily meal plan will consist of three smoothies (one for each meal), water or tea, and different healthy snacks for a consecutive ten days. This diet plan is very strict but promises healthy, dramatic weight loss (10-15 pounds in most cases) through the consumption of highly nutritious foods. While it is useful, you should not stay on this full cleanse for more than two consecutive weeks.

Approved Foods for the Full 10-Day Green Smoothie Cleanse Weight Loss Diet Plan

Ingredients for Green Smoothies:

- Choose raw foods when possible. Restrict yourself to only fruits, water, and green leafy veggies for your green smoothies.

- Opt for dark green leafy veggies like beet greens, arugula, chard/Swiss chard, carrot top leaves, dandelion greens, collard greens, radish tops, spring greens, watercress, lettuce (preferably with dark green leaves), mustard greens, spinach, sorrel, turnip greens, and similar options.

- Take off the stems from your leafy greens for better-tasting smoothie. Alternate your choice of dark leafy greens to avoid building up alkaloids.

- The composition of most green smoothies is about 40 percent protein. If you want to add more protein to fuel hard work out sessions, you can add extra protein powder to your smoothies. For this, use a single scoop of protein powder per day divided across all of your smoothies for the day to feel full for a longer time and boost your metabolism rate. Choose plant-based, non-dairy, protein powder like hemp protein, soy, or rice, instead of whey protein powder which comes from cow's milk. You can go for RAW Protein by Garden of Life, SunWarrior Protein blend, and even Rainbow Light's Acai Berry Blast Protein Energizer among other relevant options.

- Load up on fruits like seedless grapes, apples, mango, blueberries, bananas, mixed berries, pineapples, peaches, and strawberries. If you are a diabetic or have candida, choose low-sugar fruits and monitor your blood glucose levels. You should talk to your doctor before starting the 10-Day Green Smoothie Cleanse Weight Loss Diet Plan to avoid any issues that may affect your diabetes. Low-sugar fruits include grapefruits, limes, apples, cherries, lemons, cranberries, goji berries, blueberries, and strawberries. Fruits with a moderate amount of sugar consist of oranges, pears, peaches, plums, and pomegranates. High-sugar fruits include melons, papayas, mangos, apricots, kiwis, bananas, pineapples, dates, raisins, grapes, and figs. Choose to go easy on fruits and don't overdo them unnecessarily if you're concerned about your sugar levels.

- You can use either frozen or fresh fruits. However, it's always best to use ripe fruits in your smoothies. In case the fruit isn't ripe when you buy it, wait for it to get ripe before adding it to your smoothies.
- You can also use "superfoods" like acai berries or maca in your smoothies.
- Most recipes also include ground flaxseeds.
- A natural sweetener like stevia is also used in most of the smoothies.
- Opt for organic ingredients as much as possible. If you are unable to find organic ingredients, properly rinse off all the pesticides and wax from your ingredients before using them. You can use vinegar or special cleansers from health stores for this purpose.
- Always use purified water or spring water in your smoothies. You can also use alkaline water in your smoothies; this will help more in remaining hydrated and for detoxification. You can also use ice in your smoothies but tap water isn't recommended at all.

Instructions and Tips for Green Smoothies Diet Plan:

- Consume up to sixty ounces of green smoothies every day.
- Always choose smoothies instead of juices as smoothies are rich in fiber and contain whole foods.
- Try to prepare your smoothies in the morning for the entire day to save time.
- Keep the smoothies in a refrigerator until you're ready to drink them.
- Always drink a third of your smoothies throughout the day. You can also sip it whenever you feel hungry.
- If you are unable to drink the entire required amount of smoothies, drink at least 2 of them to ensure proper nutrient consumption of your body. For a revved up metabolism, drink your smoothies every 3 to 4 hours. Although you will feel less hungry, you will need energy every 4 hours or so in the form of snacks or smoothies.
- Use a high-quality blender for prepping your smoothies (i.e. 1,000 watts). Brands like Blendtec, Nutribullet, and Vitamix, etc. are all high-quality appliances. A smaller blender will require you to work in two batches to prepare your daily required smoothies.
- As a snack, you can have celery, cucumbers, apples, carrots, and various other crunchy veggies throughout the entire day.
- High-protein snacks like hard-boiled eggs, unsalted or raw nuts and seeds (a small amount), and unsweetened peanut butter, etc. are approved.
- Drink a glass or two of water in the morning to rehydrate yourself.

- Drink a cup of detox tea after the two glasses of water to cleanse and detox your kidneys and liver. You can also add stevia which is a natural sweetener for taste enhancement of your detox tea.
- You should drink plenty of water throughout the day while you are on the 10-Day Green Smoothie Cleanse Weight Loss Diet Plan. At a minimum, consume around 64 ounces or 8 glasses of water in addition to the detox tea (you can try detox tea by Yogi or Triple Leaf, etc.) or even herbal teas like green tea, peppermint tea, milk thistle tea, ginger tea, ginseng tea, sarsaparilla tea, dandelion tea, chamomile tea etc. depending on what you like.
- In the early days, you will feel irritable and hungrier. To avoid this, you can have snacks until your body adjusts to eating less during the day. However, avoid over snacking as it will impact your weight loss drastically.
- The general symptoms of detoxification are pains, cravings, nausea, headaches, irritability, skin rashes, and muscle aches. In case your detox symptoms are unbearable, follow these steps:

  - Change the fruit to veggies ratio in your smoothies. Preferably use a ratio of 30 percent veggies to 70 percent fruits and keep increasing the amount of green veggies overtime with a slight decrease in the amount of fruits you use.

  - Drink as much as water possible to strengthen the cleansing process.

  - Progress gradually in the diet plan. Have a smoothie for breakfast and have a light meal, then healthy meals for lunch and dinner on the first day of your plan. You still have to avoid dairy, meats, and sugar, etc. Then, on the second day, you can have green smoothies for both your breakfast and lunch and a light meal for your dinner. On the third day, however, you will have green smoothies for all three meals. If you are unable to do this, you can switch to the modified variation of the diet plan for the rest of the remaining days.

Foods Not Allowed on the 10-Day Green Smoothie Cleanse Weight Loss Diet Plan – Full Cleanse:

- Don't use any starchy veggies like carrots, sweet potatoes, or any other veggies not categorized as leafy greens.
- Don't use refined sugar and other products like refined carbs including sweets, white bread, and pasta.
- Avoid processed foods
- Avoid animal-based products including meat and dairy products like cheese, milk, etc.
- Avoid beverages that dehydrate you like soda (both regular and diet), beer, liquor, coffee, etc.
- Avoid fried foods.

The 10-Day Green Smoothie Cleanse Weight Loss Diet Plan – Modified Cleanse:

The modified variation of the diet plan is based on drinking two smoothies—one for breakfast and one for lunch—one healthy, natural-food meal for dinner, tea/water, and approved snacks for 10 days. This variation was specifically drafted for those who are either unable to or unwilling to commit to the full cleanse. It is also best for people who are looking more for a detox plan instead of a weight loss plan. Here, weight loss won't be as fast or dramatic but you may experience a weight loss of around 5 to 10 pounds after the 10 days.

Approved Foods for the 10-Day Green Smoothie Cleanse Weight Loss Diet Plan – Modified Cleanse:

- The same approved foods for the full cleanse plan as outlined earlier.
- Green smoothies for 2 meals every day which will weigh around 12 to 16 ounces
- A healthy meal for dinner or whatever meal you choose to replace.
- The healthy meal should have sautéed vegetables, fish, or grilled or baked chicken, and a salad, etc.
- Consume around 8 glasses or 64 ounces of water every day along with the herbal tea or detox tea.
- Drink the detox tea after consuming water in the morning.

Foods Not Allowed on the 10-Day Green Smoothie Cleanse Weight Loss Diet Plan – Modified Cleanse:

- The same as the full-cleanse plan outlined earlier.

Chapter 2: How to Continue Losing Weight After the 10-Day Challenge?

In order to continue losing weight after the 10-day plan, you need to go through the following tips and suggestions thoroughly. These are as follows:

- For continuous weight loss of about 2 pounds every week, drink two smoothies every day and a single clean meal high in protein. To lose a single pound per week, have one smoothie every day and two clean meals high in protein.
- If you hit a weight loss (no weight loss for 2 weeks) you should consider seeing a doctor to check your hormones.
- Eat a big salad consisting of a mix of dark green veggies and loads of colorful veggies.
- Consume one green leafy smoothie per day. You can also add additional protein, coconut oil, bee pollen, spirulina, and flaxseeds, for extra health benefits.
- Choose foods rich in nutrients instead of processed junk foods.
- Avoid salt, trans fats, and sugar.
- Drink plenty of pure water.
- Drink green tea and herbal teas instead of coffee.
- Eat red meat only 2 to 3 times every week.
- Eat organic ingredients as much as possible.
- Eat 4 to 5 times every day.
- Never fall to prey to emotional hunger.

You must eat protein with carbs. Each meal should comprise of double the amount of carbs in grams than the amount of protein in grams. **Supporting General Weight Loss with your Meals:**

For continued weight loss after completing the 10-day plan, eat the following foods:

1. **Animal Proteins:**
   - Poultry like skinless chicken, turkey bacon, turkey breast, Cornish hen, etc.
   - Shellfish and other seafood like clams, oysters, scallops, crabmeat, calamari, scallops, lobsters, etc.
   - Fish like flounder, halibut, sardines, catfish, bass, cod, herring, sole, wild salmon, shrimp, tuna, trout, tilapia, etc.

2. **Veggies:** Dark veggies, avocados, asparagus, Brussels sprouts, carrots, cauliflower, broccoli, collards, garlic, cucumbers, celery, collards, green beans, lettuce, olives, mushrooms, kale, onions, peas, red peppers, parsley, radishes, sweet potatoes, tomatoes, spinach, squashes, zucchini, yams, etc.

3. **Fruits:** Generally, you can have all fruits as they are healthy. But if you are looking to lose weight or have diabetes, you should eat low-sugar fruits like blueberries, blackberries, cranberries, limes, passion fruit, grapefruits, strawberries, lemons, raspberries, etc.

4. **Grains (Pasta, Rice, Bread):** Bulgur, barley, coconut flour, quinoa, brown rice, buckwheat, oats (steel cut), wild rice, etc.

5. **Legumes and Beans:** Black beans, black-eyed peas, fava beans, pinto beans, navy beans, kidney beans, garbanzo beans, chickpeas, butter beans, green beans, lima beans, lentils, white beans, etc.

6. **Dairy:** Almond milk, hemp milk, rice milk, goat's milk, coconut milk, non-dairy butter (vegan butter), eggs, egg whites.

7. **Nuts & Seeds:**
   - Unsalted and raw nuts like Brazil nuts, cedar nuts, almonds, cashews, macadamia nuts, pecans, peanuts, walnuts, pistachios, hazelnuts.

- Seeds like flaxseeds, pumpkin seeds, hemp seeds, sunflower seeds, sesame seeds, chia seeds, preferably unsalted and raw nuts, and seeds.

8. **Oils:** Coconut oil, fish oil, avocado oil, flaxseed oil, extra-virgin olive oil, and sesame oil, etc.

9. **Sweeteners:** Monk fruit agave nectar, coconut palm sugar, xylitol, stevia, raw honey, sugar alcohol, etc.

10. **Spice and Seasonings:** Black pepper, cayenne pepper, apple cider vinegar, cilantro, chili peppers, parsley, ginger, cinnamon, cardamom, nutmeg, oregano, onion, garlic, tamari, saffron, turmeric, sage, rosemary, saffron, thyme, etc.

11. **Snacks:** Popcorn (lightly salted), organic unsweetened chocolate, seeds, nuts, plain yogurt, hard-boiled eggs, trail mix, fresh veggies and fruits, unsweetened peanut butter/almond butter/cashew butter.

12. **Drinks:** Alkaline water, spring or distilled water, coconut water, black tea, green tea, herbal teas, fresh-squeezed juice, and mint tea, etc.

13. **Cooking Techniques:** Broiling, pressure cooking, sautéing, roasting, stir-frying, steaming, baking, boiling, poaching.

14. **Superfood additions for Green Smoothies:** Aloe vera, bee pollen, avocados, acai berries, chia seeds, cayenne pepper, coconut oil, flax oil, chia seeds, goji berries, ginger, brewer's yeast (nutritional), raw chocolate, maca root, sprouts, wheatgrass juice (powdered or fresh), kefir, yogurt, wheat germ (raw), pomegranate juice.

Don'ts for General Weight Loss after the 10-Day Cleanse:

Don't consume the following foods if you're looking for continued weight loss after completing the 10-day plan:

1. **Animal Protein:**
   - No processed meats like beef jerky, pepperoni, sausage, salami, bacon, hot dogs, etc.
   - High-fat meats like porterhouse, prime rib, etc.
   - Powdered eggs

2. **Veggies:** Although all veggies are considered healthy, if you are aiming for weight loss, don't eat corn, red potatoes, white potatoes, plantains, etc.

3. **Fruits:** Fried fruits, canned fruits, and fruit snacks are a no-go.

4. **Grains (Pasta, Bread, Rice):** Donuts, white flour, white pasta, bagels, white bread, etc.

5. **Legumes and Beans:** Refried beans and dried beans are considered a no-go.

6. **Dairy:** Regular cow's milk (full fat), cream cheese, sour cream, cottage cheese, cheese, condensed milk, powdered milk, yogurt (with fruit on the bottom).

7. **Nuts & Seeds:** Sugar-coated seeds and nuts.

8. **Oils:** Margarine, vegetable oils, trans fats (hydrogenated oils), chicken fat, and bacon fat.

9. **Sweeteners:** High fructose corn syrup (HFCS), brown sugar, brown rice syrup, raw sugar, fruit juice concentrate, dextrose, white sugar.

10. **Seasonings & Spices:** MSG, mayonnaise, ketchup, Worcestershire sauce, table salt.

11. **Snacks:** Corn chips, cakes, potato chips, cookies, candies, donuts, pies, ice cream pastries.

12. **Drinks:** Sports drinks, beer, mixed drinks, sodas, store-bought fruit juices

13. **Cooking methods:** Barbequing, burning, charring, pan frying, deep frying, blackening.

Pros of the 10-Day Green Smoothie Cleanse Weight Loss Diet Plan:

1. Easy and convenient diet plan for just 10 days.
2. Can help out in detoxification and in overcoming cravings and food addiction.
3. Effective weight loss ranging from 10 to 15 pounds in just days.
4. Based on natural foods.
5. Keeps your body healthy and maintained.

Cons of the 10-Day Green Smoothie Cleanse Weight Loss Diet Plan:

1. You might experience irritation, fatigue, and other detox symptoms in the early stages.
2. Many foods are excluded from your diet including pasta, potatoes, alcohol, legumes, caffeine, cereal, bread, and fruit.
3. Expensive and costly due to additional protein supplements in the smoothies.
4. Organic foods are required which might also increase the cost of the entire diet plan.

Chapter 3: The 10-Day Green Smoothie Meal Plan

Day 1

Breakfast Smoothie: Turmeric Ginger Detox Smoothie

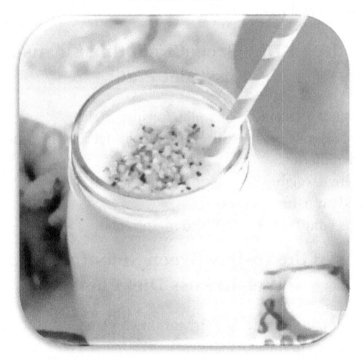

Preparation time: 10 minutes
Total time: 10 minutes
Servings: 2

Ingredients:

- 1 yellow squash, chopped
- 1 orange, peeled

- 2 tbsp kumquats
- ½ tsp turmeric
- ½ inch ginger , peeled
- 1 tbsp hemp seed
- 1 cup water
- 1 cup ice

How to prepare:

1. Add all ingredients in a blender except squash and ice.
2. Now blend the mixture until smooth.
3. Add in squash and blend again.
4. Add ice and blend again.
5. Pour into serving glasses and enjoy.

Nutritional Values:
Calories 85
Total Fat 3 g
Saturated Fat 0 g
Cholesterol 0 mg
Sodium 0 mg
Total Carbs 14 g
Fiber 3 g
Sugar 8 g
Protein 1.5 g

Lunch Smoothie: Apple Chia Detox Smoothie

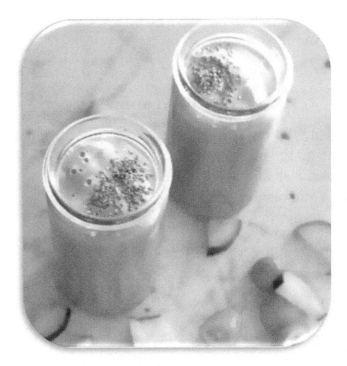

Preparation time: 10 minutes
Total time: 10 minutes
Servings: 2

Ingredients:

- 3 tbsp collard greens
- 1 mini cucumber, chopped
- 4 kumquats
- 1 apple, chopped
- ½ tsp chlorella
- 1 tbsp chia seeds
- 1 cup water
- 1 cup ice

How to prepare:

1. Add all ingredients in a blender and mix until smooth.
2. Pour into serving glasses and enjoy.

Nutritional Values:
Calories 108
Total Fat 2 g
Saturated Fat 0 g
Cholesterol 0 mg
Sodium 0 mg
Total Carbs 21 g
Fiber 9 g
Sugar 11 g
Protein 3 g

Dinner Smoothie: Almond Avocado Matcha Smoothie

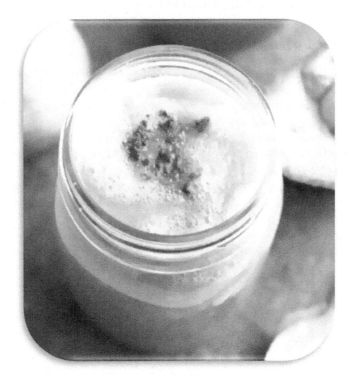

Preparation time: 10 minutes
Total time: 10 minutes
Servings: 2

Ingredients:

- 3 tbsp red lettuce
- 1 pear, chopped
- ½ avocado, pitted
- 1 tsp Matcha
- 1 tbsp almond butter
- 1 cup vanilla almond milk
- 1 cup ice

How to prepare:

1. Add all ingredients in a blender except ice.
2. Now blend the mixture until smooth.
3. Add in ice and blend again.
4. Pour into serving glasses and enjoy.
5. You can add more ice if you want your smoothie to be more chilled.

Nutritional Values:
Calories 178
Total Fat 11 g
Saturated Fat 0 g
Cholesterol 0 mg
Sodium 10 mg
Total Carbs 20 g
Fiber 8 g
Sugar 9 g
Protein 3 g

Day 2

Breakfast Smoothie: Sweet Potato Smoothie

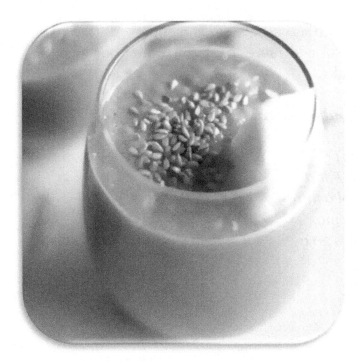

Preparation time: 10 minutes
Total time: 10 minutes
Servings: 2

Ingredients:

- 10 tbsp sweet potato, scrubbed, chopped
- 8 tbsp pineapple, chopped
- 1 orange, peeled
- 1 tbsp flaxseed
- ½ tsp camu camu powder
- 1 cup water
- 1 cup ice

How to prepare:

1. Add all ingredients to a blender.
2. Blend until you reach smoothness you desire.
3. Pour the smoothie into serving glasses.
4. Serve and enjoy!

Nutritional Values:

Calories 140
Total Fat 2 g
Saturated Fat 0 g
Cholesterol 0 mg
Sodium 0 mg
Total Carbs 32 g
Fiber 6 g
Sugar 15 g
Protein 3 g

Lunch Smoothie: Banana Oatmeal Detox Smoothie

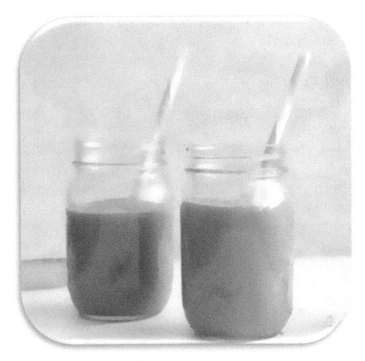

Preparation time: 10 minutes
Total time: 10 minutes
Servings: 2

Ingredients:

- 3 tbsp collard greens
- 1 banana, peeled
- 1 apple, chopped
- 3 tbsp, oats
- 1 tsp cinnamon
- 1 cup water
- 1 cup ice

How to prepare:

1. Add all ingredients except ice in a blender.
2. Now blend the mixture until smooth.
3. Add in ice and blend again.
4. Pour into serving glasses and enjoy.

Nutritional Values:
Calories 162
Total Fat 1 g
Saturated Fat 0 g
Cholesterol 0 mg
Sodium 0 mg
Total Carbs 41 g
Fiber 14 g
Sugar 13 g
Protein 3 g

Dinner Smoothie: Rhubarb Detox Smoothie

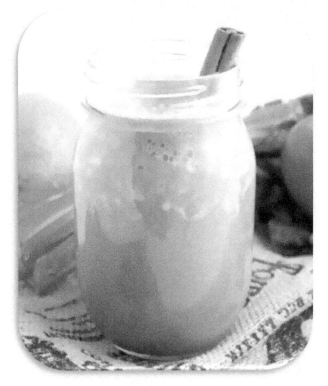

Preparation time: 10 minutes
Total time: 10 minutes
Servings: 2

Ingredients:

- 3 tbsp Swiss chard
- 1 orange, peeled
- ¼ cup rhubarb, chopped
- ½ tsp cinnamon
- 1 tbsp hemp protein
- 1 cup water
- 1 cup ice

How to prepare:

1. Place all ingredients except ice in a blender.
2. Now blend the mixture until smooth.
3. Add in ice and blend again.
4. Pour into serving glasses and enjoy.

Nutritional Values:
Calories 76
Total Fat 1 g
Saturated Fat 0 g
Cholesterol 0 mg
Sodium 0 mg
Total Carbs 17 g
Fiber 7 g
Sugar 7 g
Protein 3 g

Day 3

Breakfast Smoothie: Apple Celery Detox Smoothie

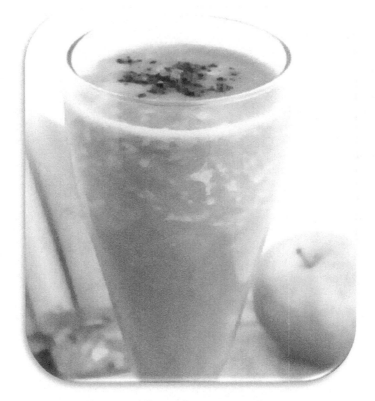

Preparation time: 10 minutes
Total time: 10 minutes
Servings: 2

Ingredients:

- 3 tbsp collard greens
- 2 ribs celery
- 1 apple, chopped

- 3 sprigs mint
- 2 tbsp raw hazelnuts
- ½ tsp moringa
- 1 cup water
- 1 cup ice

How to prepare:

1. Add all ingredients in a blender.
2. Now blend the mixture until smooth.
3. Pour into serving glasses and enjoy.

Nutritional Values:
Calories 115
Total Fat 5 g
Saturated Fat 0 g
Cholesterol 0 mg
Sodium 0 mg
Total Carbs 14 g
Fiber 6 g
Sugar 10 g
Protein 3 g

Lunch Smoothie: Zucchini Detox Smoothie

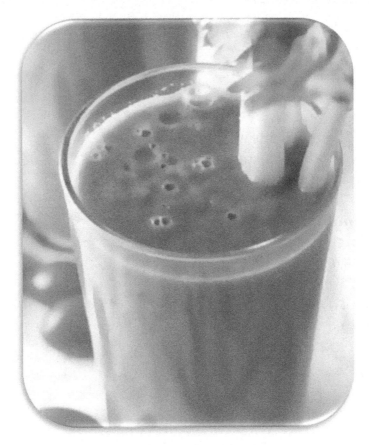

Preparation time: 10 minutes
Total time: 10 minutes
Servings: 2

Ingredients:

- 1 zucchini
- 8 tbsp grape tomatoes
- 6 tbsp celery stocks
- 1 tbsp sea beans
- ½ jalapeno pepper, seeded

- ½ lemon, juiced
- 1 tsp maqui berry powder
- 1 cup water
- 1 cup ice

How to prepare:

1. Add all ingredients except zucchini into a blender.
2. Add zucchini and blend the mixture until smooth.
3. Pour into serving glasses and enjoy.

Nutritional Values:
Calories 50
Total Fat 0.5 g
Saturated Fat 0 g
Cholesterol 0 mg
Sodium 0 mg
Total Carbs 10 g
Fiber 3 g
Sugar 4 g
Protein 2.4 g

Dinner Smoothie: Purple Detox Smoothie

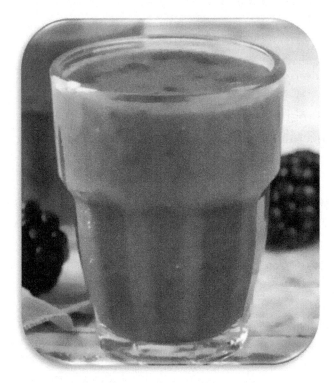

Preparation time: 10 minutes
Total time: 10 minutes
Servings: 2

Ingredients:

- 2 tbsp blackberries
- 4 tbsp pineapple, chopped
- 1 apple, chopped
- 2 sprigs sage
- ½ tsps maqui berry powder
- 2 tbsp walnuts
- 1 cup water
- 1 cup ice

How to prepare:

1. Add all ingredients to a blender.
2. Now blend the mixture until smooth.
3. Pour into serving glasses and enjoy.

Nutritional Values:

Calories 143
Total Fat 6 g
Saturated Fat 0 g
Cholesterol 0 mg
Sodium 0 mg
Total Carbs 23 g
Fiber 10 g
Sugar 11 g
Protein 5 g

Day 4

Breakfast Smoothie: Carrot Detox Smoothie

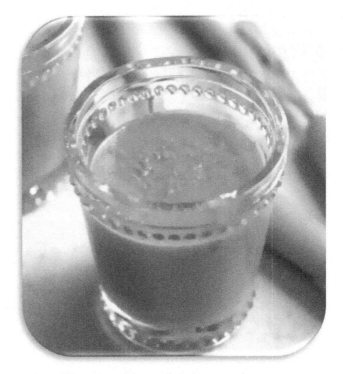

Preparation time: 10 minutes
Total time: 10 minutes
Servings: 2

Ingredients:

- 10 tbsp carrot, chopped
- 1 banana, peeled
- 1 inch ginger, peeled and chopped
- 1 inch turmeric peeled, chopped
- 1 tsp cinnamon
- 1 cup coconut milk
- 1 cup ice

How to prepare:

1. Add all ingredients to a blender.
2. Now blend the mixture until smooth.
3. Pour into serving glasses and enjoy your drink.

Nutritional Values:
Calories 134
Total Fat 3 g
Saturated Fat 0 g
Cholesterol 0 mg
Sodium 0 mg
Total Carbs 30 g
Fiber 12 g
Sugar 9 g
Protein 2 g

Lunch Smoothie: Rhubarb Citrus Detox Smoothie

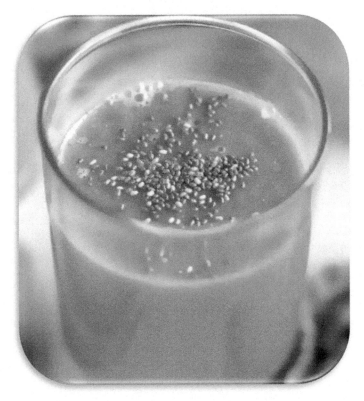

Preparation time: 10 minutes
Total time: 10 minutes
Servings: 2

Ingredients:

- 3 tbsp Swiss chard
- 8 tbsp cantaloupe
- 1 pear, chopped
- 4 tbsp rhubarb, chopped
- 1 lime, peeled

- 1 tbsp chia seeds
- 1 cup water
- 1 cup ice

How to prepare:

1. Add all ingredients to a blender.
2. Now blend the mixture until smooth.
3. You can add more ice if you want your drink to be more chilled.
4. Pour into serving glasses and enjoy.

Nutritional Values:
Calories 109
Total Fat 2 g
Saturated Fat 0 g
Cholesterol 0 mg
Sodium 0 mg
Total Carbs 23 g
Fiber 7 g
Sugar 12 g
Protein 3 g

Dinner Smoothie: Blueberry Avocado Detox Smoothie

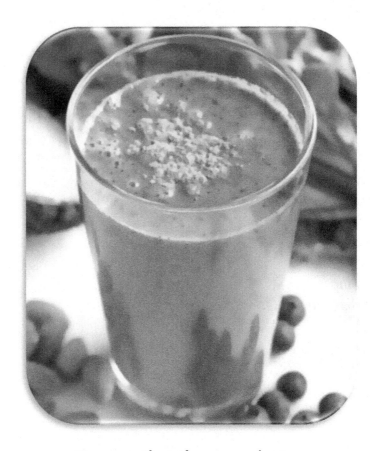

Preparation time: 10 minutes
Total time: 10 minutes
Servings: 2

Ingredients:

- 3 tbsp Swiss chard
- ½ avocado, pitted
- 1 pear, chopped
- 4 tbsp blueberries

- 2 tbsp almonds
- ½ tsp camu camu
- 1 cup water
- 1 cup ice

How to prepare:

1. Add all ingredients to a blender.
2. Now blend the mixture until smooth.
3. Pour into serving glasses and enjoy.

Nutritional Values:

Calories 200
Total Fat 12 g
Saturated Fat 0 g
Cholesterol 10 mg
Sodium 0 mg
Total Carbs 23 g
Fiber 8 g
Sugar 11 g
Protein 4 g

Day 5

Breakfast Smoothie: Pear Jicama Detox Smoothie

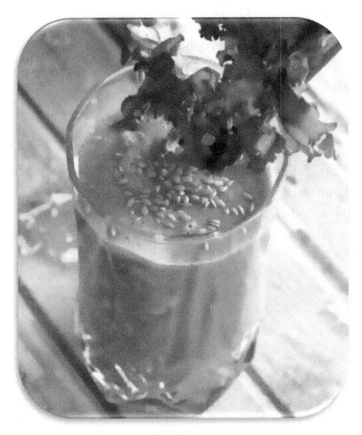

Preparation time: 10 minutes
Total time: 10 minutes
Servings: 2

Ingredients:

- 3 tbsp red kale
- 1 pear, chopped

- 8 tbsp jicama, peeled and chopped
- 1 lemon, juiced
- 1 tsp reishi mushroom
- 1 tbsp flaxseed
- 1 cup water
- 1 cup ice

How to prepare:

1. Add all ingredients to a blender.
2. Now blend the mixture until smooth.
3. Pour into serving glasses and enjoy.

Nutritional Values:
Calories 102
Total Fat 0 g
Saturated Fat 0.1 g
Cholesterol 0 mg
Sodium 0 mg
Total Carbs 24 g
Fiber 8 g
Sugar 10 g
Protein 2 g

Lunch Smoothie: Coconut Pineapple Detox Smoothie

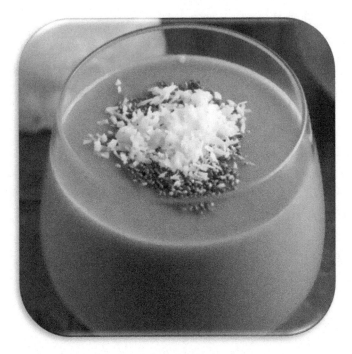

Preparation time: 10 minutes
Total time: 10 minutes
Servings: 2

Ingredients:

- 3 tbsp Swiss chard
- 8 tbsp pineapple, chopped
- 1 orange, peeled
- ½ avocado, pitted
- 2 tbsp coconut flakes
- 1 tbsp chia seeds
- 1 cup water
- 1 cup ice

How to prepare:

1. Add all ingredients to a blender.
2. Now blend the mixture until smooth.
3. Pour into serving glasses and enjoy.

Nutritional Values:
Calories 212
Total Fat 0 g
Saturated Fat 0 g
Cholesterol 0 mg
Sodium 0.2 mg
Total Carbs 26 g
Fiber 9 g
Sugar 12 g
Protein 3 g

Dinner Smoothie: Ginger Apple Detox Smoothie

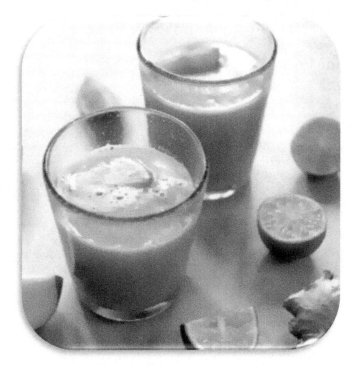

Preparation time: 10 minutes
Total time: 10 minutes
Servings: 2

Ingredients:

- 1 squash, chopped
- 1 apple, chopped
- 1 lime, juiced
- ½ inch ginger
- 1 tsp camu camu powder
- 1 tbsp pea protein
- 1 cup water
- 1 cup ice

How to prepare:

1. Add all ingredients except ginger into a blender.
2. Now blend the mixture until smooth.
3. Add in ginger and again blend until desired consistency is reached.
4. Pour into serving glasses and enjoy.

Nutritional Values:
Calories 83
Total Fat 0 g
Saturated Fat 0 g
Cholesterol 0 mg
Sodium 0 mg
Total Carbs 19 g
Fiber 44 g
Sugar 9 g
Protein 5 g

Day 6

Breakfast Smoothie: Zesty Orange Smoothie

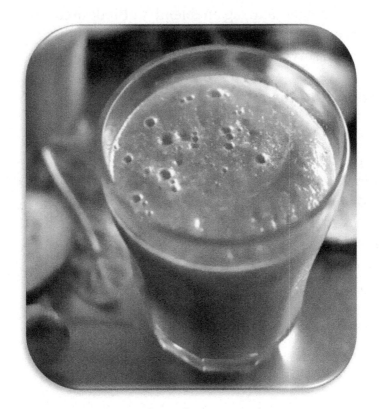

Preparation time: 10 minutes
Total time: 10 minutes
Servings: 2

Ingredients:

- 3 tbsp baby spinach
- 1 cucumber, chopped
- 1 apple, chopped
- 1 orange, peeled
- 1 lime, peeled

- 1 tbsp flaxseed
- 1 cup water
- 1 cup ice

How to prepare:

1. Add all ingredients to a blender.
2. Now blend the mixture until smooth.
3. Pour into serving glasses and enjoy.

Nutritional Values:
Calories 113
Total Fat 2 g
Saturated Fat 0 g
Cholesterol 0 mg
Sodium 0 mg
Total Carbs 27 g
Fiber 7 g
Sugar 15 g
Protein 2 g

Lunch Smoothie: Ginger Cantaloupe Detox Smoothie

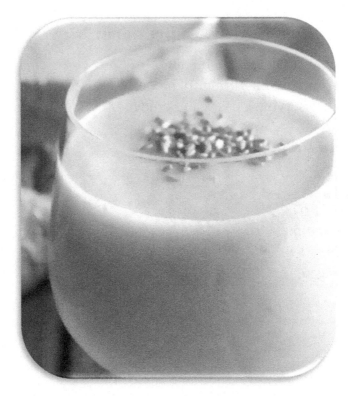

Preparation time: 10 minutes
Total time: 10 minutes
Servings: 2

Ingredients:

- 1 slice cantaloupe
- 1 pear, chopped
- ½ inch ginger, peeled
- 1 tbsp flaxseed
- 1 cup water
- 1 cup ice

How to prepare:

1. Add all ingredients except ginger to a blender.
2. Now blend the mixture until smooth.
3. Add in ginger and blend again.
4. Pour into serving glasses and enjoy.

Nutritional Values:
Calories 85
Total Fat 2 g
Saturated Fat 0 g
Cholesterol 0 mg
Sodium 0.5 mg
Total Carbs 19 g
Fiber 4 g
Sugar 12 g
Protein 2 g

Dinner Smoothie: Orange Cider Detox Smoothie

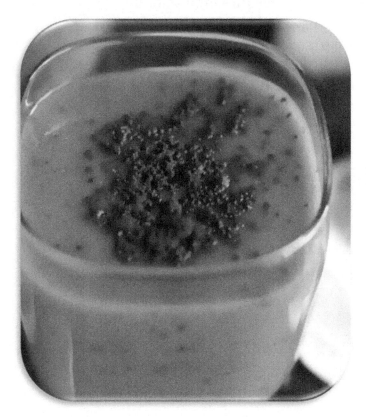

Preparation time: 10 minutes
Total time: 10 minutes
Servings: 2

Ingredients:

- 3 tbsp collard greens
- 2 clementines, peeled
- ½ avocado, pitted
- 1 tbsp apple cider vinegar
- ½ lemon, juiced

- 1 tbsp pea protein
- ¼ tsp ground cloves
- 1 cup water
- 1 cup ice

How to prepare:

1. Add all ingredients except apple cider vinegar to a blender.
2. Now blend the mixture until smooth.
3. Add apple cider vinegar in the end and give it a stir.
4. Pour into serving glasses and enjoy.

Nutritional Values:
Calories 136
Total Fat 6 g
Saturated Fat 0 g
Cholesterol 0 mg
Sodium 0 mg
Total Carbs 17 g
Fiber 6 g
Sugar 8 g
Protein 8 g

Day 7

Breakfast Smoothie: Cranberry Detox Smoothie

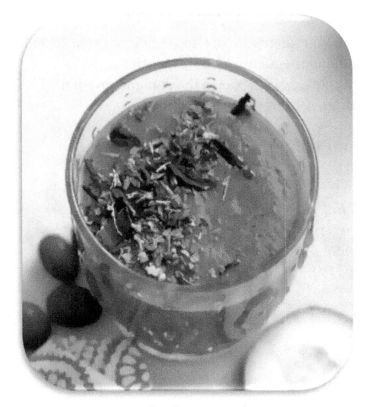

Preparation time: 10 minutes
Total time: 10 minutes
Servings: 2

Ingredients:

- 3 tbsp collard greens
- 1 apple, chopped
- 4 tbsp cranberries

- 1 mini cucumber, chopped
- 1 tbsp dried hibiscus
- 1 tbsp flaxseed
- 1 cup water
- 1 cup ice

How to prepare:

1. Add all ingredients to a blender.
2. Now blend the mixture until smooth.
3. Pour the smoothie into serving glasses and enjoy.

Nutritional Values:
Calories 89
Total Fat 1 g
Saturated Fat 0 g
Cholesterol 0 mg
Sodium 0 mg
Total Carbs 20 g
Fiber 7 g
Sugar 10 g
Protein 1 g

Lunch Smoothie: Orange Turmeric Smoothie

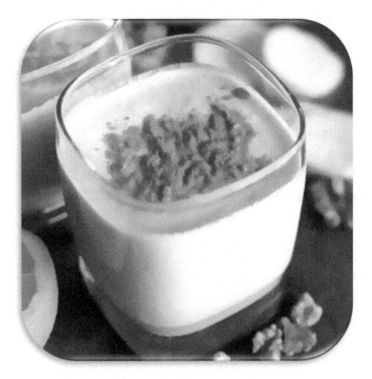

Preparation time: 10 minutes
Total time: 10 minutes
Servings: 2

Ingredients:

- 1 banana, peeled
- 1 orange, peeled
- 8 tbsp pineapple, chopped
- 3 tbsp walnuts
- 1 inch turmeric
- 1 cup water
- 1 cup ice

How to prepare:

1. Add all ingredients to a blender.
2. Now blend the mixture until smooth.
3. Pour the smoothie into serving glasses and enjoy.

Nutritional Values:

Calories 145
Total Fat 8 g
Saturated Fat 0 g
Cholesterol 0 mg
Sodium 0 mg
Total Carbs 19 g
Fiber 0 g
Sugar 13 g
Protein 3 g

Dinner Smoothie: Beet Detox Smoothie

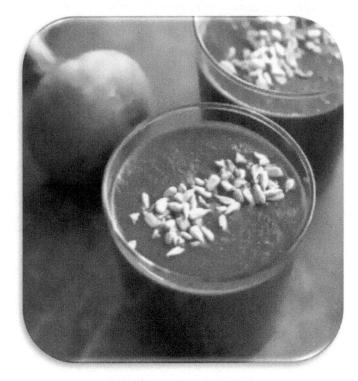

Preparation time: 10 minutes
Total time: 10 minutes
Servings: 2

Ingredients:

- 3 tbsp baby spinach
- 8 tbsp beets scrubbed, chopped
- 1 pear, chopped
- ½ inch ginger
- 1 lemon, juiced
- 1 tbsp sunflower seeds
- 1 cup water
- 1 cup ice

How to prepare:

1. Add all ingredients to a blender.
2. Now blend the mixture until smooth.
3. Pour the mixture into serving glasses and enjoy!

Nutritional Values:

Calories 99
Total Fat 2 g
Saturated Fat 0 g
Cholesterol 0 mg
Sodium 0 mg
Total Carbs 20 g
Fiber 4 g
Sugar 12 g
Protein 3 g
Potassium 0 mg

Day 8

Breakfast Smoothie: Chamomile Ginger Detox Smoothie

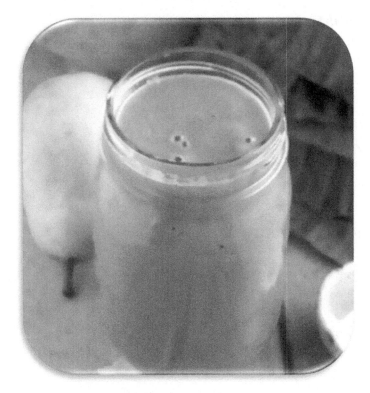

Preparation time: 10 minutes
Total time: 10 minutes
Servings: 2

Ingredients:

- 3 tbsp collard greens
- 1 pear, chopped
- 1 slice cantaloupe, chopped
- ½ lemon, juiced

- ½ inch ginger, peeled
- 1 tbsp dried chamomile flowers
- 1 cup water
- 1 cup ice

How to prepare:

1. Place all ingredients in a blender.
2. Now blend the mixture until smooth.
3. Serve and enjoy!

Nutritional Values:
Calories 86
Total Fat 0 g
Saturated Fat 0 g
Cholesterol 0 mg
Sodium 0 mg
Total Carbs 22 g
Fiber 4 g
Sugar 15 g
Protein 2 g

Lunch Smoothie: Dill Detox Smoothie

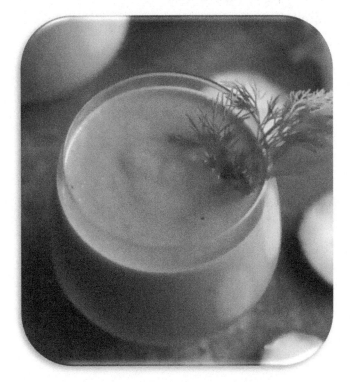

Preparation time: 10 minutes
Total time: 10 minutes
Servings: 2

Ingredients:

- 3 tbsp baby spinach
- 2 cucumbers, chopped
- 1 pear, chopped
- 1 lime, juiced
- 2 sprigs dill
- 1 tsp pomegranate powder
- 1 cup water
- 1 cup ice

How to prepare:

1. Add all ingredients except dill into a blender.
2. Now blend the mixture until smooth.
3. Add in dill and blend again.
4. Pour into serving glasses, serve and enjoy.

Nutritional Values:

Calories 85
Total Fat 0.3 g
Saturated Fat 0 g
Cholesterol 0 mg
Sodium 0 mg
Total Carbs 22 g
Fiber 6 g
Sugar 8 g
Protein 1.4 g

Dinner Smoothie: Ginger Beet Detox Smoothie

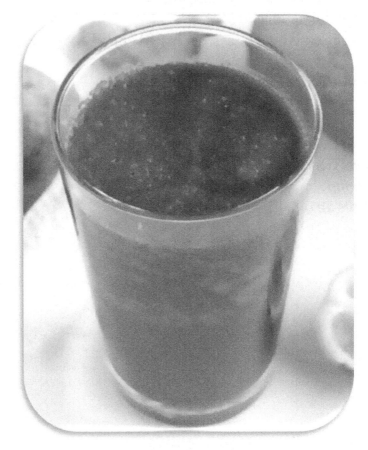

Preparation time: 10 minutes
Total time: 10 minutes
Servings: 2

Ingredients:

- 8 tbsp beets, chopped
- 4 tbsp mango, sliced
- 1 lemon, peeled

- ½ tsp wheatgrass
- ½ inch ginger
- 1 cup water
- 1 cup ice

How to prepare:

1. Place all ingredients in a blender.
2. Now blend the mixture until smooth.
3. Pour into serving glasses and enjoy.

Nutritional Values:

Calories 42
Total Fat 0 g
Saturated Fat 0 g
Cholesterol 0 mg
Sodium 0 mg
Total Carbs 10 g
Fiber 2 g
Sugar 7 g
Protein 1 g

Day 9

Breakfast Smoothie: Wheatgrass Detox Smoothie

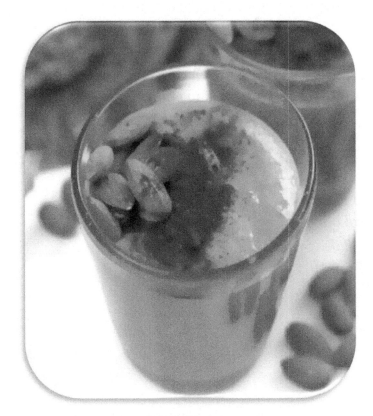

Preparation time: 10 minutes
Total time: 10 minutes
Servings: 2

Ingredients:

- 3 tbsp Swiss chard
- 2 kiwis, peeled
- 1 banana, peeled

- 3 tbsp almonds
- 1 tsp wheatgrass powder
- 1 cup water
- 1 cup ice

How to prepare:

1. Add all ingredients except kiwis in a blender.
2. Now blend the mixture until smooth.
3. Add kiwis and blend again.
4. Pour into serving glasses and enjoy.

Nutritional Values:
Calories 154
Total Fat 6 g
Saturated Fat 0 g
Cholesterol 0 mg
Sodium 0 mg
Total Carbs 24 g
Fiber 5 g
Sugar 13 g
Protein 4 g

Lunch Smoothie: Charcoal Lemonade Detox Smoothie

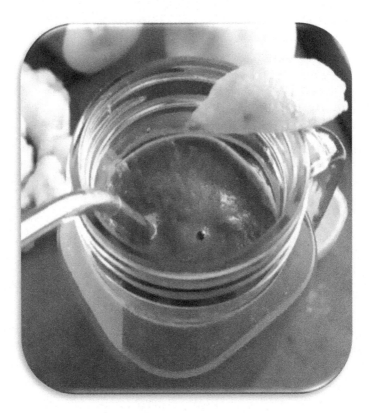

Preparation time: 10 minutes
Total time: 10 minutes
Servings: 2

Ingredients:

- 3 tbsp collard greens
- 1 apple, chopped
- 1 cucumber, chopped
- 1 lemon, peeled
- ½ inch ginger

- ½ tsp activated charcoal
- 1 cup water
- 1 cup ice

How to prepare:

1. Add all ingredients in a blender.
2. Blend until the desired consistency is reached.
3. Pour into serving glasses and enjoy.
4. You can add more ice if you prefer.

Nutritional Values:
Calories 88
Total Fat 0.6 g
Saturated Fat 0 g
Cholesterol 0 mg
Sodium 0 mg
Total Carbs 23 g
Fiber 4.6 g
Sugar 12 g
Protein 2 g

Dinner Smoothie: Orange Detox Smoothie

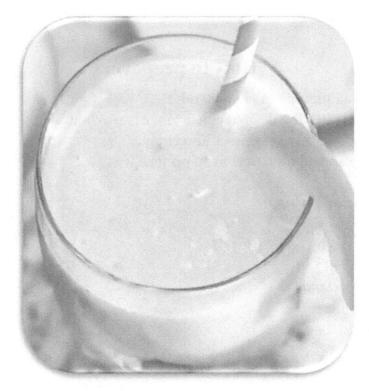

Preparation time: 10 minutes
Total time: 10 minutes
Servings: 1

Ingredients:

- 1/3 cup almond milk
- 3 large oranges, peeled
- ½ tsp pure vanilla extract
- ½ tsp vanilla powdered protein
- 1 cup ice

How to prepare:

1. Place all ingredients in a blender.
2. Blend until the texture is smooth.
3. Pour into serving glasses and enjoy.

Nutritional Values:

Calories 499
Total Fat 20 g
Saturated Fat 17 g
Cholesterol 5 mg
Sodium 49 mg
Total Carbs 70.6 g
Fiber 15 g
Sugar 55.1 g
Protein 18.5 g
Potassium 1,240 mg

Day 10

Breakfast Smoothie: Blueberry Kale Smoothie

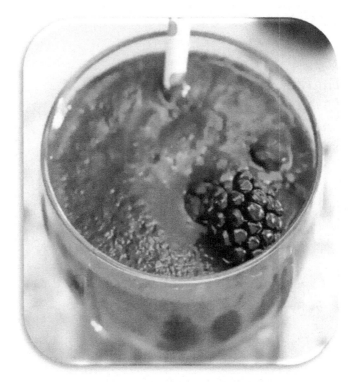

Preparation time: 10 minutes
Total time: 10 minutes
Servings: 1

Ingredients:

- ½ cup coconut water
- ½ cup kale
- 5 fresh blackberries
- 2 cups frozen blueberries
- 1 cup frozen pineapple chunks

How to prepare:

1. Place all ingredients in a blender.
2. Blend until the texture is smooth.
3. Pour into serving glasses and enjoy.
4. You can add more coconut water to make it thinner.

Nutritional Values:

Calories 395
Total Fat 1.3 g
Saturated Fat 0 g
Cholesterol 0 mg
Sodium 25 mg
Total Carbs 100.4 g
Fiber 10.5 g
Sugar 80.7 g
Protein 4.3 g

Lunch Smoothie: Raspberry Strawberry Detox Smoothie

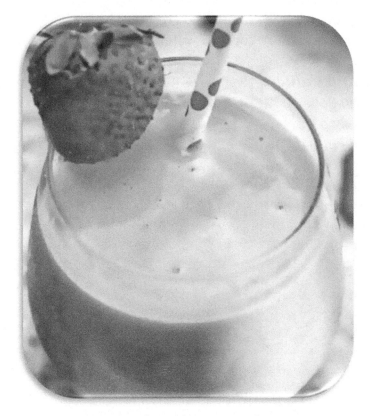

Preparation time: 10 minutes
Total time: 10 minutes
Servings: 1

Ingredients:

- 2 cups frozen strawberries, sliced
- 1 cup frozen mango chunks
- 4-5 fresh raspberries
- 1/3 cup coconut cream
- 1 cup coconut water

How to prepare:

1. In a high speed blender, add all ingredients and add ½ cup of coconut water.
2. Blend until it is smooth.
3. Add in remaining coconut water and blend again.
4. Pour into serving glasses and enjoy.

Nutritional Values:

Calories 469
Total Fat 20.2 g
Saturated Fat 17.4 g
Cholesterol 0 mg
Sodium 265 mg
Total Carbs 74.7 g
Fiber 19.7 g
Sugar 52 g
Protein 4.7 g

Dinner Smoothie: Peach Detox Smoothie

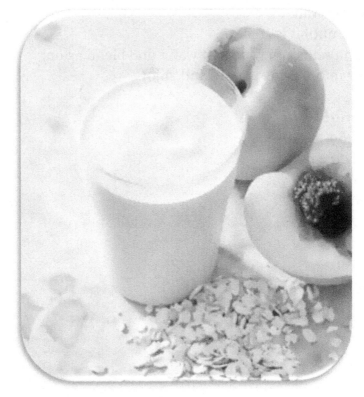

Preparation time: 10 minutes
Total time: 10 minutes
Servings: 1

Ingredients:

- 1 cup frozen peach slices
- 1 cup Greek yogurt
- ¼ cup oatmeal
- ¼ tsp vanilla extract
- 1 cup almond milk

How to prepare:

1. In a high speed blender, add all ingredients except peach slices.
2. Blend until it is smooth.
3. Add in peach slices and blend again.
4. Pour into serving glasses and enjoy.

Nutritional Values:

Calories 331
Total Fat 4 g
Saturated Fat 0 g
Cholesterol 0 mg
Sodium 0 mg
Total Carbs 46 g
Fiber 5 g
Sugar 12 g
Protein 29 g

Chapter 4: Detox Green Smoothies Recipes For Weight Loss

Basic Green Banana Smoothie

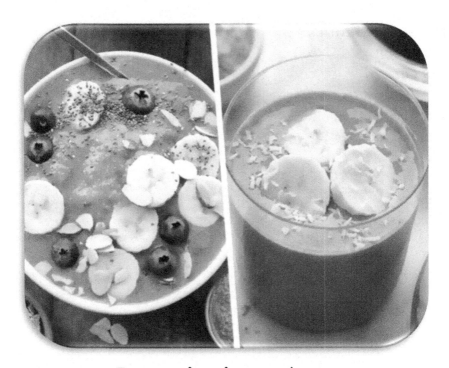

Preparation time: 5 minutes
Total time: 5 minutes
Servings: 1

Ingredients:

- 1 cup frozen banana
- 1 cup frozen blueberries
- 1 cup spinach
- 1 cup almond milk
- ½ tbsp chia seeds

How to prepare:

Place all ingredients into a blender and mix until smooth.

Note: It is good to begin with ½ cup of milk and then add rest of the ingredients.

Nutritional Values:

Calories 146
Total Fat 3 g
Saturated Fat 0 g
Cholesterol 0 mg
Sodium 0.21 mg
Total Carbs 30 g
Fiber 5 g
Sugar 14 g
Protein 3 g

Peanut Green Smoothie

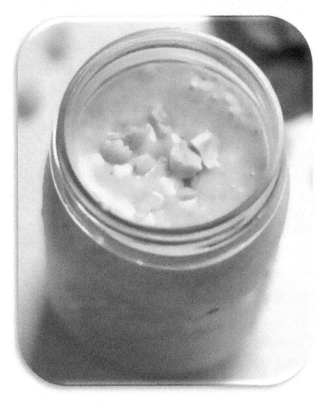

Preparation time: 5 minutes
Total time: 5 minutes
Servings: 1

Ingredients:

- 1 medium banana, ripe
- 1 tbsp peanut butter
- 2 tbsp peanuts, salted
- 1 cup almond milk
- 1 handful of spinach
- 6 large ice cubes

How to prepare:

1. Add all ingredients into a blender and blend until smooth.
2. Pour into serving glasses and enjoy.

Nutritional Values:
Calories 326
Total Fat 15 g
Saturated Fat 0 g
Cholesterol 0 mg
Sodium 0 mg
Total Carbs 43 g
Fiber 0 g
Sugar 23 g
Protein 10 g

Tropical Spinach Green Smoothie

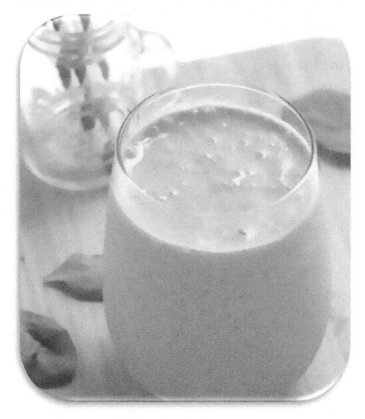

Preparation time: 5 minutes
Total time: 5 minutes
Servings: 1

Ingredients:

- 2 cups tropical blend frozen fruit
- ½ cup full-fat canned coconut milk
- ½ cup water
- 2 cups packed fresh spinach
- 1 tbsp ground flaxseed

How to prepare:

1.   Add all ingredients to a blender.
2.   Blend until smooth.
3.   Serve and enjoy!
4.   You can use ice if you want more chilled smoothie.

Nutritional Values:

Calories 203
Total Fat 11 g
Saturated Fat 0 g
Cholesterol 0 mg
Sodium 45 mg
Total Carbs 22 g
Fiber 5 g
Sugar 15 g
Protein 3 g

Pineapple Kale Green Smoothie

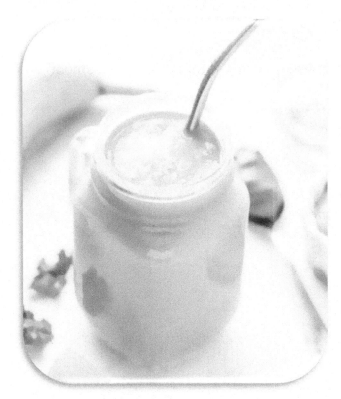

Preparation time: 10 minutes
Total time: 10 minutes
Servings: 1

Ingredients:

- 2 cups kale leaves, chopped
- ¾ cup almond milk
- 1 frozen medium banana, chopped
- ¼ cup plain, non-fat Greek yogurt
- ¼ cup frozen pineapple pieces
- 2 tbsp peanut butter
- Honey, to taste

How to prepare:

1. Add all ingredients to a high-speed blender.
2. Blend until desired consistency is reached.
3. Pour into serving glasses and enjoy your drink.

Nutritional Values:
Calories 187
Total Fat 9 g
Saturated Fat 1 g
Cholesterol 3 mg
Sodium 149 mg
Total Carbs 27 g
Fiber 4 g
Sugar 13 g
Protein 8 g

Protein Green Detox Smoothie

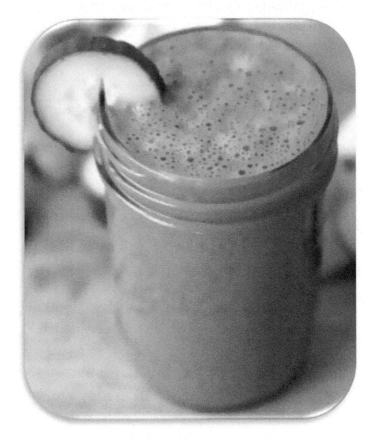

Preparation time: 10 minutes
Total time: 10 minutes
Servings: 1

Ingredients:

- ½ cup unsweetened almond milk
- 1 tbsp almond butter
- 1 banana, chopped
- 2 cups spinach

How to prepare:

1.   Add all ingredients to a blender.
2.   Blend until it is smooth.
3.   Pour into serving glasses and enjoy.

Nutritional Values:

Calories 237
Total Fat 11.4 g
Saturated Fat 1 g
Cholesterol 0 mg
Sodium 140 mg
Total Carbs 33.1 g
Fiber 6.5 g
Sugar 15.4 g
Protein 6.9 g

Kiwi Detox Green Smoothie

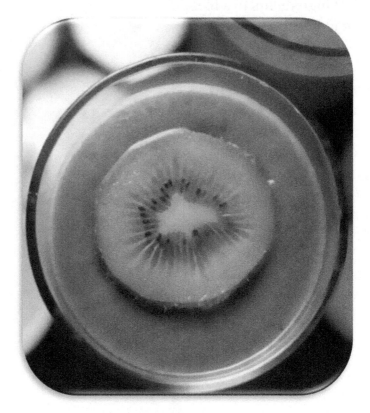

Preparation time: 10 minutes
Total time: 10 minutes
Servings: 1

Ingredients:

- 1 kiwi
- 1 banana
- ¼ cup pineapple
- 2 celery stalks
- 2 cups spinach
- 1 cup water

How to prepare:

1. Add all ingredients to a blender.
2. Blend until it is smooth.
3. Pour into serving glasses and enjoy.

Nutritional Values:

Calories 191
Total Fat 1.1 g
Saturated Fat 0.2 g
Cholesterol 0 mg
Sodium 86 mg
Total Carbs 46.7 g
Fiber 7.8 g
Sugar 26 g
Protein 4.3 g

Apple Berry Spinach Smoothie

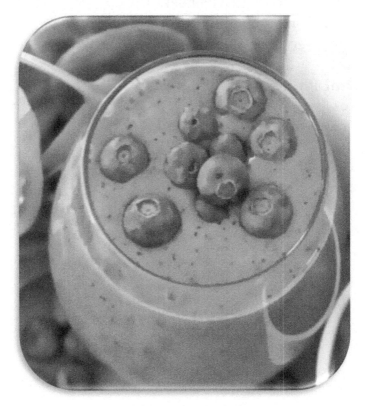

Preparation time: 10 minutes
Total time: 10 minutes
Servings: 1

Ingredients:

- ½ cup strawberries
- ½ cup raspberries
- 1 large apple
- 2 cups spinach
- 1 cup water

How to prepare:

1. Add all ingredients to a blender.
2. Blend until desired consistency is reached.
3. Serve and enjoy!

Nutritional Values:

Calories 185
Total Fat 1.3 g
Saturated Fat 0.1 g
Cholesterol 0 mg
Sodium 58 mg
Total Carbs 45.9 g
Fiber 12.2 g
Sugar 29.7 g
Protein 3.5 g

Pineapple Banana Green Detox Smoothie

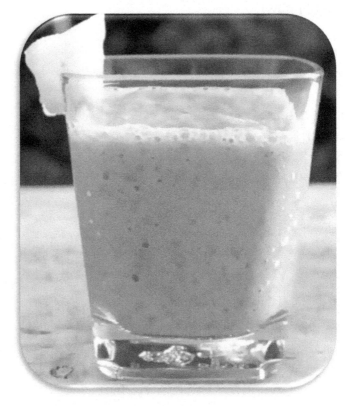

Preparation time: 10 minutes
Total time: 10 minutes
Servings: 1

Ingredients:

- 1 cup pineapple, chopped
- 1 banana, chopped
- 1 apple, chopped
- 2 cups spinach
- 1 cup water

How to prepare:

1. Add all ingredients to a blender.
2. Blend until desired consistency is reached.
3. Serve and enjoy!

Nutritional Values:

Calories 317
Total Fat 1.2 g
Saturated Fat 0.2 g
Cholesterol 0 mg
Sodium 60 mg
Total Carbs 81.6 g
Fiber 12.1 g
Sugar 54.1 g
Protein 4.5 g

Kale and Apple Green Detox Smoothie

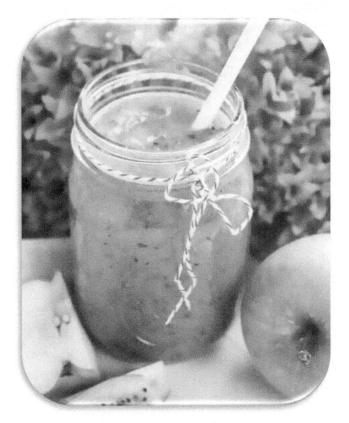

Preparation time: 10 minutes
Total time: 10 minutes
Servings: 1

Ingredients:

- ⅔ cup almond milk
- ¾ cup ice
- 1 ½ cups kale, chopped
- 1 stalk celery, chopped
- ½ apple, chopped and cored
- 1 tbsp ground flaxseed

How to prepare:

1. Add all ingredients to a blender.
2. Blend until desired consistency is reached.
3. Serve and enjoy!
4. You can add more ice if you want.

Nutritional Values:

Calories 515
Total Fat 40.6 g
Saturated Fat 34.1 g
Cholesterol 0 mg
Sodium 89 mg
Total Carbs 37.3 g
Fiber 9.9 g
Sugar 17.3 g
Protein 8.4 g

Kale Strawberry Banana Detox Smoothie

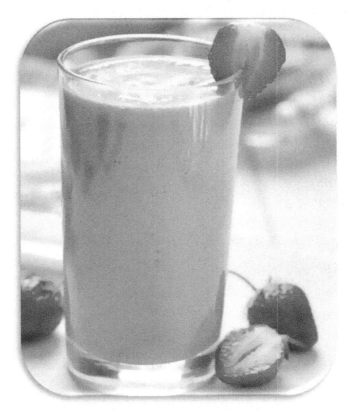

Preparation time: 10 minutes
Total time: 10 minutes
Servings: 1

Ingredients:

- 1 banana
- 1 cup yogurt
- 1 cup strawberries
- 1 cup Kale, chopped
- 1 cup ice

How to prepare:

1. Place all ingredients in a blender.
2. Blend until smooth.
3. Pour into serving glasses and enjoy.
4. You can add water if you want your smoothie to be thinner.

Nutritional Values:

Calories 358
Total Fat 3.8 g
Saturated Fat 2.6 g
Cholesterol 15 mg
Sodium 210 mg
Total Carbs 62.3 g
Fiber 7 g
Sugar 38.7 g
Protein 18.2 g

Parsley and Cucumber Green Detox Smoothie

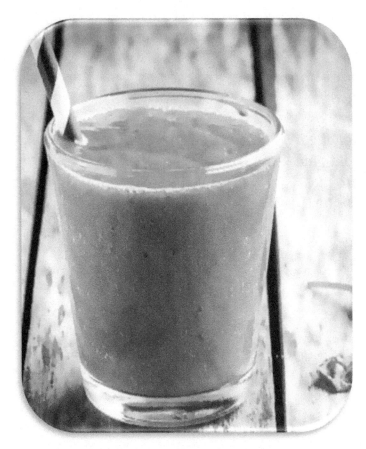

Preparation time: 10 minutes
Total time: 10 minutes
Servings: 2

Ingredients:

- 1 cucumber, chopped
- 1 inch ginger root, chopped
- 1 cup parsley

- 1 lemon, juiced
- 1 cup spinach
- ½ orange, sliced
- 1 cup ice cubes
- 1 cup coconut cream
- 2 cups water

How to prepare:

1. Place all ingredients in a blender.
2. Blend until it is smooth.
3. Pour into serving glasses and enjoy.

Nutritional Values:

Calories 164
Total Fat 14.6 g
Saturated Fat 12.8 g
Cholesterol 0 mg
Sodium 28 mg
Total Carbs 8.8 g
Fiber 2.4 g
Sugar 4.5 g
Protein 2.7 g

Blackberries Ginger Green Detox Smoothie

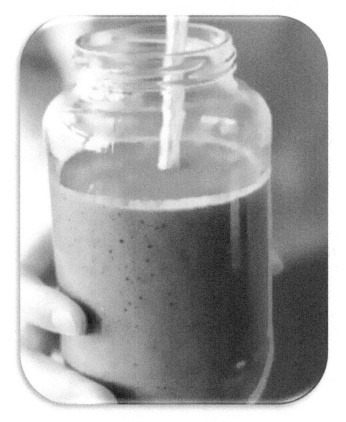

Preparation time: 10 minutes
Total time: 10 minutes
Servings: 6

Ingredients:

- 1 cup romaine lettuce
- 4 cups water
- 1/3 cup blackberries
- 1 tbsp fresh ginger, peeled and chopped

- 1 cup raw cucumber, peeled and sliced
- ½ avocado, cubed
- 2 tbsp fresh parsley
- 4 tbsp lemon juice
- 1 pack coconut butter
- 1 tbsp granulated Swerve

How to prepare:

1. Place all ingredients in avocado blender.
2. Blend until it is smooth.
3. Pour into serving glasses and enjoy.

Nutritional Values:

Calories 231
Total Fat 7 g
Saturated Fat 4 g
Cholesterol 0 mg
Sodium 5 mg
Total Carbs 5.4 g
Fiber 2.9 g
Sugar 1.4 g
Protein 1.1 g

Chocolate Green Detox Smoothie

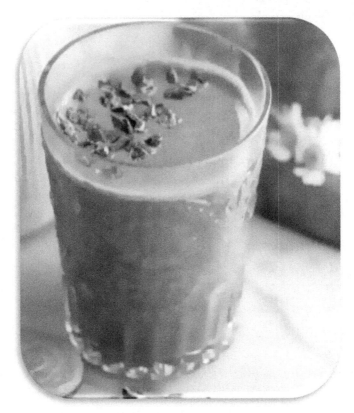

Preparation time: 10 minutes
Total time: 10 minutes
Servings: 4

Ingredients:

- 1 cup coconut cream
- ½ cup fresh raspberries
- 2 cups water
- 2 cups spinach, chopped
- 2 tbsp stevia
- ¼ cup cocoa powder

How to prepare:

1. Place all ingredients except cocoa powder in a blender.
2. Blend until it is smooth.
3. Add in cocoa powder and blend again.
4. Pour into serving glasses and enjoy.

Nutritional Values:

Calories 161
Total Fat 15.2 g
Saturated Fat 13.1 g
Cholesterol 0 mg
Sodium 26 mg
Total Carbs 8.7 g
Fiber 4.3 g
Sugar 2.8 g
Protein 3 g

Green Lemon Detox Smoothie

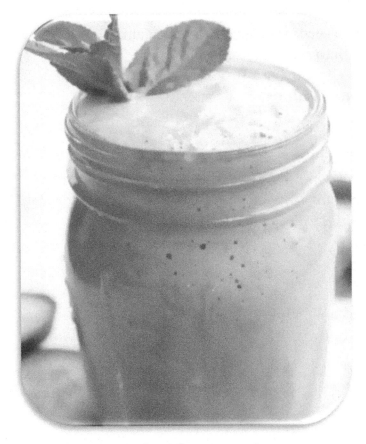

Preparation time: 10 minutes
Total time: 10 minutes
Servings: 4

Ingredients:

- ½ cucumber
- ½ large avocado
- 3 tbsp lemon juice
- ½ cup coconut milk
- 2 cups water

- 1 scoop hemp protein powder
- 1 cup ice
- 3 drops lemon essential oil
- 2 cups organic baby spinach leaves, lightly steamed
- 1 tbsp coconut oil
- 1 scoop pumpkin seed protein powder
- 1 tbsp Xylitol

How to prepare:

1. Place all ingredients except protein powders into a blender.
2. Blend until it is smooth.
3. Add protein powders and blend on low.
4. Pour into serving glasses and enjoy.

Nutritional Values:
Calories 208
Total Fat 16.9 g
Saturated Fat 10.6 g
Cholesterol 0 mg
Sodium 24 mg
Total Carbs 8 g
Fiber 4.2 g
Sugar 2.2 g
Protein 8.6 g

Avocado and Mint Green Detox Smoothie

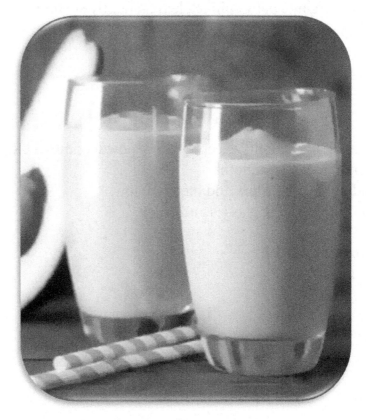

Preparation time: 10 minutes
Total time: 10 minutes
Servings: 3

Ingredients:

- 1½ cups full-fat coconut milk
- 1 avocado, chopped
- 1 cup almond milk
- 10 large mint leaves

- 1 tbsp lime juice
- 2 cups crushed ice
- 1 cup water
- 1 scoop stevia
- 6 cilantro sprigs
- ½ tsp vanilla extract

How to prepare:

1. Place all ingredients except ice in a blender.
2. Puree until smooth.
3. Add ice and blend on low.
4. Pour into serving glasses.

Nutritional Values:
Calories 303
Total Fat 30.4 g
Saturated Fat 22.5 g
Cholesterol 0 mg
Sodium 20 mg
Total Carbs 9.1 g
Fiber 4.8 g
Sugar 3.6 g
Protein 3.2 g

Coconut Green Smoothie

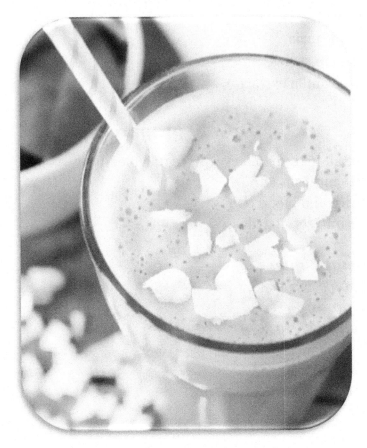

Preparation time: 10 minutes
Total time: 10 minutes
Servings: 2

Ingredients:

- 2 tbsp ground flaxseed
- 1 cup Swiss chard, chopped
- 1 cup raw spinach
- ¼ cup strawberries
- ¼ cup coconut, shredded

- 2 tsp ginger, grated
- 1 tsp lemon juice
- 1 tbsp coconut oil
- 10 ice cubes

How to prepare:

1. Place all ingredients in a blender.
2. Blend until it is smooth.
3. Pour into serving glasses and enjoy.

Nutritional Values:
Calories 157
Total Fat 12.7 g
Saturated Fat 9.2 g
Cholesterol 0 mg
Sodium 64 mg
Total Carbs 8.4 g
Fiber 4.7 g
Sugar 2 g
Protein 3.5 g

Low-Carb Green Detox Smoothie

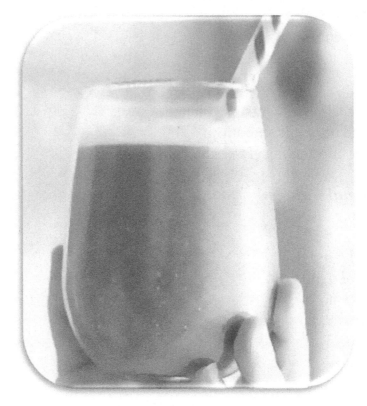

Preparation time: 10 minutes
Total time: 10 minutes
Servings: 6

Ingredients:

- 4 tbsp spinach
- ½ cup celery
- 2 cups almond milk
- 1 small cucumber
- 1 cup ice
- 1 cup water

- ½ avocado
- 2 tbsp coconut oil
- 1 scoop pumpkin seeds protein powder
- 1 tsp Matcha powder
- 10 drops liquid stevia

How to prepare:

1. Add all ingredients except ice to a blender.
2. Blend until it is smooth.
3. Add in ice and blend again.
4. Pour into serving glasses and enjoy.
5. You can garnish it with chia seeds if you want.

Nutritional Values:
Calories 298
Total Fat 27.8 g
Saturated Fat 21.7 g
Cholesterol 0 mg
Sodium 42 mg
Total Carbs 10.3 g
Fiber 4.9 g
Sugar 3.9 g
Protein 6.3 g

Mint Green Protein Detox Smoothie

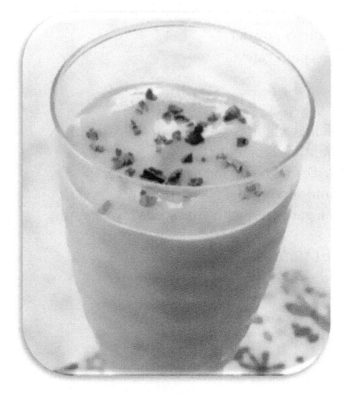

Preparation time: 10 minutes
Total time: 10 minutes
Servings: 2

Ingredients:

- 1 cup fresh spinach
- 1 scoop hemp protein powder
- ½ avocado
- 8 drops liquid stevia
- ½ cup unsweetened almond milk
- ½ cup ice
- ¼ tsp peppermint extract

How to prepare:

1. Put spinach, avocado, almond milk and protein powder in a blender and blend until smooth.
2. Add in all remaining ingredients and blend again.
3. Serve and enjoy.

Nutritional Values:

Calories 209
Total Fat 12.6 g
Saturated Fat 2.5 g
Cholesterol 0 mg
Sodium 65 mg
Total Carbs 7.7 g
Fiber 5.6 g
Sugar 0.6 g
Protein 5.6 g

Coconut Mint Green Detox Smoothie

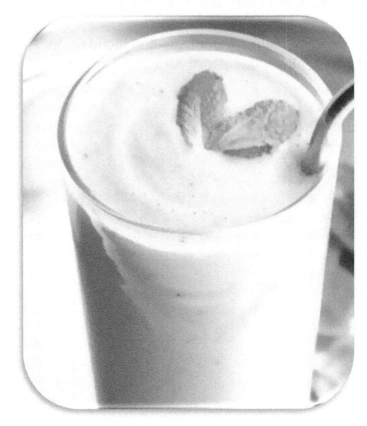

Preparation time: 10 minutes
Total time: 10 minutes
Servings: 4

Ingredients:

- 24 tbsp water
- 3 scoops hemp protein powder
- 4 tbsp mint, chopped
- 4 tbsp coconut oil
- ¼ tsp sea salt

- 16 tbsp full-fat milk
- 1 cup frozen cauliflower
- 1 avocado, chopped
- 4 tsp vanilla extract
- ¼ tsp cinnamon
- Coconut flakes, for garnish

How to prepare:

1. Put all ingredients in a blender.
2. Blend until smooth.
3. Garnish with coconut flakes and serve.

Nutritional Values:
Calories 214
Total Fat 33.9 g
Saturated Fat 23.3 g
Cholesterol 0 mg
Sodium 149 mg
Total Carbs 10.2 g
Fiber5.8 g
Sugar 2.7 g
Protein 8.1 g

Green Olives Detox Smoothie

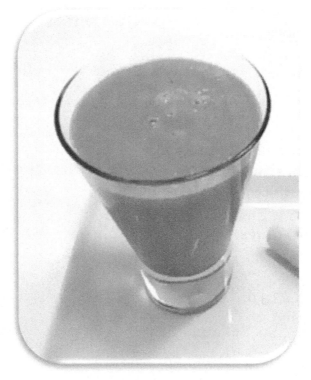

Preparation time: 10 minutes
Total time: 10 minutes
Servings: 2

Ingredients:

- 2 cups fresh spinach
- ¼ cup coconut, peeled
- 1 cup water
- 1½ cups full-fat coconut milk
- 1 cup raspberries
- 1 cup crushed ice
- ½ cup green olives
- 2 tbsp ground flaxseed

How to prepare:

1. Add spinach, coconut, water, raspberries, green olives, coconut milk, and flaxseed to a blender and blend until smooth.
2. Add ice and blend again.
3. Serve chilled and enjoy.

Nutritional Values:

Calories 293
Total Fat 27 g
Saturated Fat 20.7 g
Cholesterol 0 mg
Sodium 409 mg
Total Carbs 11 g
Fiber 5.7 g
Sugar 4.8 g
Protein 3.7 g

Jalapeno Green Detox Smoothie

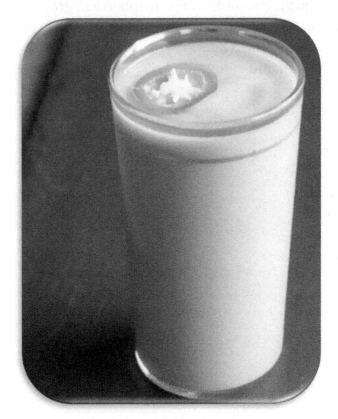

Preparation time: 10 minutes
Total time: 10 minutes
Servings: 2

Ingredients:

- 2 cups baby spinach
- 1 cup blackberries
- 1 cup full-fat coconut milk
- 1 avocado, chopped
- 1½ cups water
- ½ tsp jalapeno pepper, chopped

How to prepare:

1. Add spinach, blackberries, coconut milk, avocado, water and jalapeno to a blender.
2. Blend until smooth.
3. Serve and enjoy.
4. You can garnish with jalapeno pepper on top.

Nutritional Values:

Calories 193
Total Fat 17.6 g
Saturated Fat 10.5 g
Cholesterol 0 mg
Sodium 24 mg
Total Carbs 8.3 g
Fiber 4.5 g
Sugar 2.5 g
Protein 2.3 g

Green Tea Pear Detox Smoothie

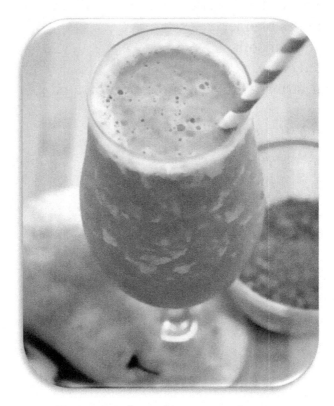

Preparation time: 10 minutes
Total time: 10 minutes
Servings: 4

Ingredients:

- 1 scoop pea protein powder
- 1½ cups almond milk
- 1 cup fresh spinach
- 1 cup water
- ½ pear, cored
- ½ tsp green tea powder
- 2 tbsp cashews, chopped

How to prepare:

1. Place all the ingredients except protein powder in a blender.
2. Blend until smooth.
3. Add protein powder and blend again.
4. Serve and enjoy!

Nutritional Values:

Calories 826
Total Fat 81.2 g
Saturated Fat 70.2 g
Cholesterol 0 mg
Sodium 141 mg
Total Carbs 22.9 g
Fiber 8.4 g
Sugar 13 g
Protein 14.7 g

Pineapple Detox Green Smoothie

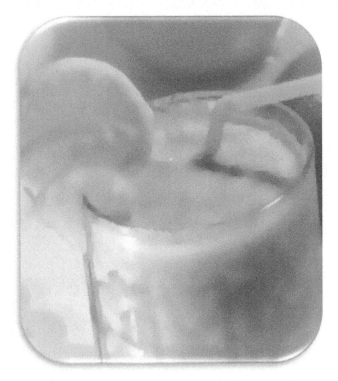

Preparation time: 5 minutes
Total time: 5 minutes
Servings: 3

Ingredients:

- 2 cups fresh spinach
- 2 oranges, peeled
- 1 cup water
- 1 cup red seedless grapes
- 1 cup crushed ice
- ½ cup fresh pineapple, chopped
- 2 tbsp ground flaxseed

How to prepare:

1. Add spinach, oranges, water, grapes and pineapple to a blender.
2. Blend until smooth.
3. Add ice and flaxseeds and blend again.
4. Serve and enjoy.

Nutritional Values:

Calories 175
Total Fat 4.4 g
Saturated Fat 1.4 g
Cholesterol 7 mg
Sodium 38 mg
Total Carbs 33.1 g
Fiber 7.4 g
Sugar 23.3 g
Protein 4.4 g

Citrus Green Detox Smoothie

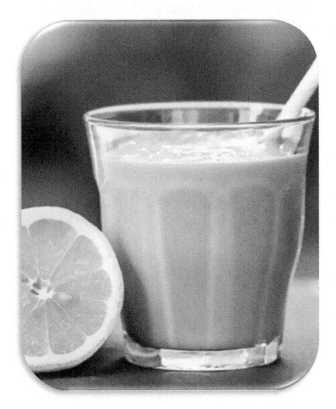

Preparation time: 10 minutes
Total time: 10 minutes
Servings: 2

Ingredients:

- 2 cups almond milk
- 2 oranges
- 2 tbsp lime juice
- 2 tsp orange zest
- 2 handfuls spinach
- 2 tbsp lemon juice
- 2 cups ice

How to prepare:

1. Put all the ingredients in a blender and blend.
2. Serve and enjoy.

Nutritional Values:

Calories 657
Total Fat 57.7 g
Saturated Fat 50.9 g
Cholesterol 0 mg
Sodium 51 mg
Total Carbs 39.7 g
Fiber 10.2 g
Sugar 26.3 g
Protein 7.6 g

Cucumber Ginger Detox Smoothie

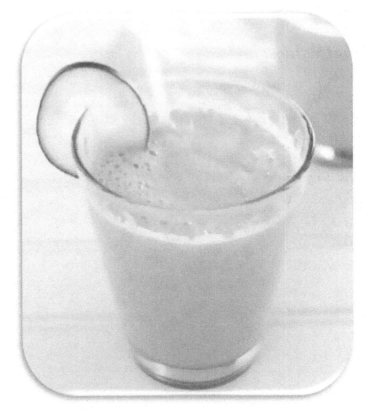

Preparation time: 10 minutes
Total time: 10 minutes
Servings: 4

Ingredients:

- 1½ cups water
- 1 lemon, juiced
- ¼ avocado, pitted and peeled
- 1 cup baby spinach
- ½ cup cucumber, chopped
- 2 tbsp hemp seeds

- ½ tsp ground ginger
- Sea salt, to taste
- 1 cup ice cubes

How to prepare:

1. Add all ingredients to a blender.
2. Blend for 35 seconds.
3. Serve chilled and enjoy!

Nutritional Values:
Calories 78
Total Fat 6 g
Saturated Fat 0.7 g
Cholesterol 0 mg
Sodium 76 mg
Total Carbs 4.5 g
Fiber 1.8 g
Sugar 0.7 g
Protein 3.2 g

Peach Green Smoothie

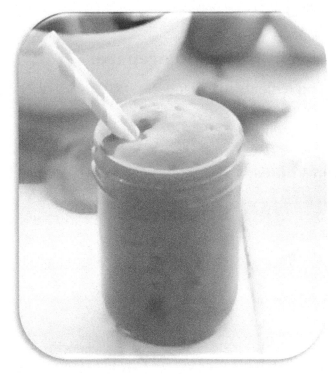

Preparation time: 10 minutes
Total time: 10 minutes
Servings: 2

Ingredients:

- ½ cup almond milk
- 1 cup baby spinach
- 1 medium banana
- ¾ cup frozen peach chunks
- ½ lemon, juiced
- 1 tbsp chia seeds

How to prepare:

1. Add all ingredients to a blender.
2. Blend until smooth.
3. Pour into serving glasses and enjoy.

Nutritional Values:

Calories 151
Total Fat 3 g
Saturated Fat 2 g
Cholesterol 0 mg
Sodium 52 mg
Total Carbs 31 g
Fiber 6 g
Sugar 18 g
Protein 3 g

Peach Walnut Green Smoothie

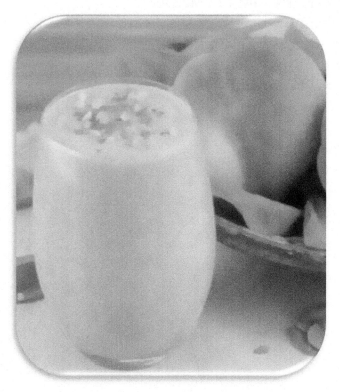

Preparation time: 10 minutes
Total time: 10 minutes
Servings: 1

Ingredients:

- 1 peach, sliced (fresh or frozen)
- ¼ cup walnuts, chopped
- ¼ tsp cinnamon
- 1 tsp coconut oil
- 1 cup spinach, packed
- ½ cup water
- 4 ice cubes

How to prepare:

1. Add all ingredients to a blender.
2. Blend until desired consistency is reached.
3. Serve and enjoy.

Nutritional Values:

Calories 300
Total Fat 23.5 g
Saturated Fat 5 g
Cholesterol 0 mg
Sodium 28 mg
Total Carbs 18.7 g
Fiber 5.4 g
Sugar 14.5 g
Protein 9.8 g

Calorie Burning Green Smoothie

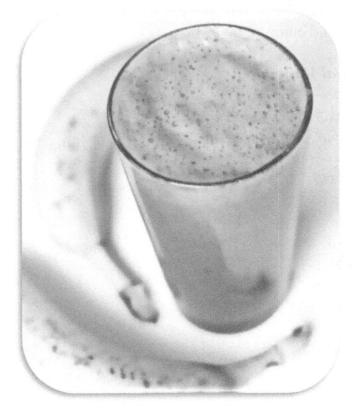

Preparation time: 10 minutes
Total time: 10 minutes
Servings: 1

Ingredients:

- 1 cup baby spinach
- 1 ripe banana
- 1 cup almond milk
- 1 cup frozen pineapple chunks
- ½ tsp ginger
- 1 tbsp chia seeds

How to prepare:

1. Add all ingredients to a blender.
2. Blend until smooth.
3. Serve chilled and enjoy.

Nutritional Values:

Calories 1,049
Total Fat 66.6 g
Saturated Fat 51.8 g
Cholesterol 0 mg
Sodium 207 mg
Total Carbs 117.2 g
Fiber 25.9 g
Sugar 74.2 g
Protein 14.5 g

Cucumber Mint Detox Green Smoothie

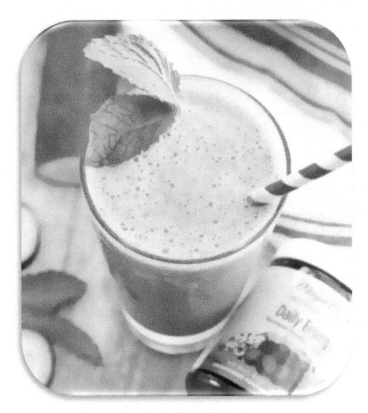

Preparation time: 10 minutes
Total time: 10 minutes
Servings: 1

Ingredients:

- 1 cucumber, sliced
- ¼ cup almond milk
- 3 large mint leaves
- 1 scoop *Mega Food Daily Energy Nutrient Booster Powder*
- ½ tsp pure stevia powder
- 1 cup ice

How to prepare:

1.   Add all the ingredients to a blender.
2.   Blend until smooth.
3.   Serve chilled and have fun!

Nutritional Values:

Calories 183
Total Fat 14.6 g
Saturated Fat 12.8 g
Cholesterol 0 mg
Sodium 22 mg
Total Carbs 14.3 g
Fiber 2.9 g
Sugar 7 g
Protein 3.3 g

Matcha Mango Green Smoothie

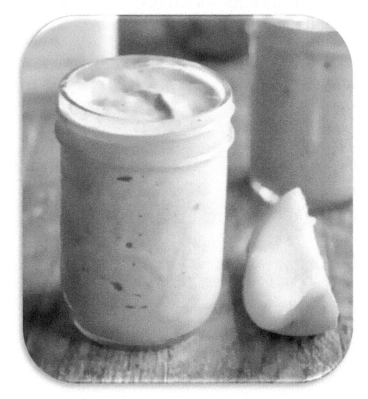

Preparation time: 5 minutes
Total time: 5 minutes
Servings: 1

Ingredients:

- ½ avocado, chopped
- ½ tsp Matcha green tea
- ½ cup mango, cubed
- 1 cup baby greens
- 1 cup almond milk
- Stevia, to taste

How to prepare:

1. Add all ingredients to a blender.
2. Blend for 35 seconds.
3. Add more stevia if needed, blend again for 5 seconds.
4. Serve chilled and enjoy!

Nutritional Values:
Calories 887
Total Fat 77.1 g
Saturated Fat 54.9 g
Cholesterol 0 mg
Sodium 213 mg
Total Carbs 49.4 g
Fiber 16.3 g
Sugar 20.9 g
Protein 12.1 g

Ginger Goddess Detox Smoothie

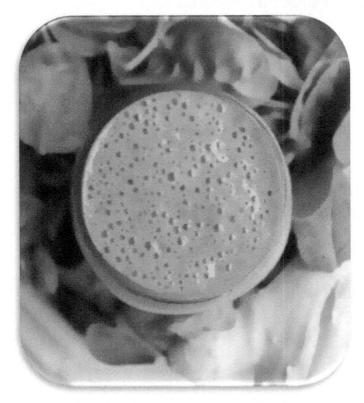

Preparation time: 10 minutes
Total time: 10 minutes
Servings: 1

Ingredients:

- 1 cup organic spinach
- 2 pieces organic celery
- ½ avocado, chopped
- 1 chunk fresh ginger
- ½ cup almond milk
- 1 cup ice

How to prepare:

1. Add all the ingredients to a blender.
2. Blend until smooth.
3. Serve chilled!

Nutritional Values:

Calories 535
Total Fat 48.4 g
Saturated Fat 29.5 g
Cholesterol 0 mg
Sodium 255 mg
Total Carbs 27.7 g
Fiber 14.2 g
Sugar 4.8 g
Protein 7.7 g

Green Spirulina Smoothie

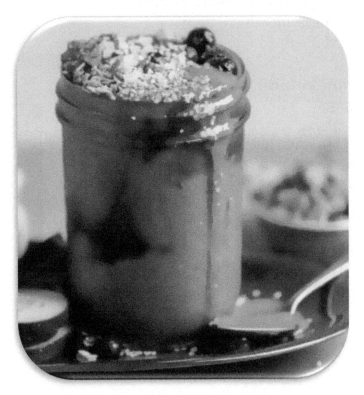

Preparation time: 10 minutes
Total time: minutes
Servings: 1

Ingredients:

- 1 medium ripe banana
- ½ cup cucumber, sliced
- 1 cup coconut milk
- 1 cup spinach
- 1 tsp spirulina powder
- 1 tbsp hemp seed

How to prepare:

1. Add all the ingredients to a blender.
2. Blend until smooth.
3. Serve chilled and enjoy.

Nutritional Values:

Calories 225
Total Fat 9.7 g
Saturated Fat 8.7 g
Cholesterol 0 mg
Sodium 72 mg
Total Carbs 36.8 g
Fiber 4 g
Sugar 15.4 g
Protein 5.8 g

Chia Seed Green Detox Smoothie

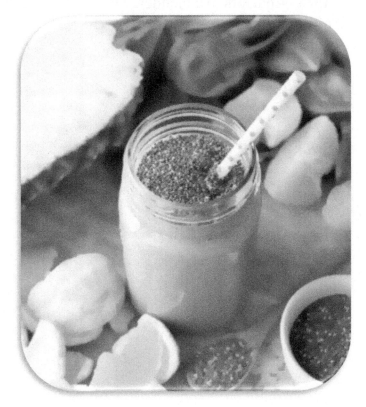

Preparation time: 10 minutes
Total time: 10 minutes
Servings: 2

Ingredients:

- 2 cups spinach
- 1 cup water
- 2 oranges, peeled
- 1 cup pineapple
- 2 tbsp chia seeds

How to prepare:

1. Add all the ingredients to a blender.
2. Blend until smooth.
3. Pour into serving glasses and enjoy.

Nutritional Values:
Calories 272
Total Fat 9.1 g
Saturated Fat 1 g
Cholesterol 0 mg
Sodium 33 mg
Total Carbs 45.5 g
Fiber 16 g
Sugar 25.5 g
Protein 7.7 g

Green Detox Burst

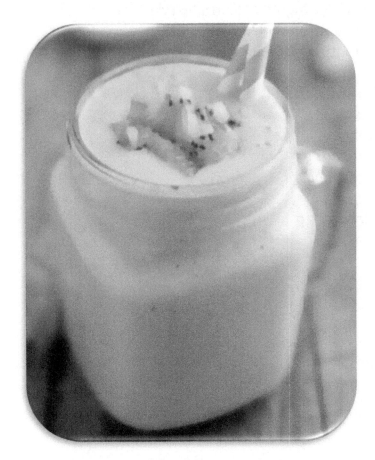

Preparation time: 10 minutes
Total time: 10 minutes
Servings: 1

Ingredients:

- ¾ cup plain Greek yogurt
- 1 scoop protein powder
- ½ cup green grapes
- 1 kiwi, peeled

- 1 banana, peeled
- 1 green apple, cored
- ½ cup pineapple, chopped
- ½ cup kale, stems removed
- 6 ice cubes

How to prepare:

1. Add all ingredients except kiwi and protein powder to a blender.
2. Blend until desired consistency is reached.
3. Add kiwi and protein powder.
4. Blend for 30 seconds and serve chilled.

Nutritional Values:
Calories 544
Total Fat 3.5 g
Saturated Fat 1.3 g
Cholesterol 67 mg
Sodium 179 mg
Total Carbs 104.2 g
Fiber 12.8 g
Sugar 70.4 g
Protein 33.7 g

Feijoada Green Detox Smoothie

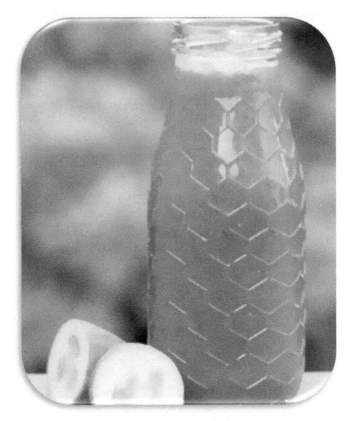

Preparation time: 10 minutes
Total time: 10 minutes
Servings: 2

Ingredients:

- 1 ripe banana
- 1 apple, cored and chopped
- 4 feijoada, flesh scooped
- 2 cups spinach
- Juice of one lime
- 1 cup water

How to prepare:

1. Add all ingredients to the blender.
2. Blend until desired consistency is reached.
3. Serve chilled.

Nutritional Values:

Calories 160
Total Fat 0.8 g
Saturated Fat 0.2 g
Cholesterol 0 mg
Sodium 0 mg
Total Carbs 40.6 g
Fiber 9.8 g
Sugar 0 g
Protein 0.8 g

Pear Kiwi Detox Green Smoothie

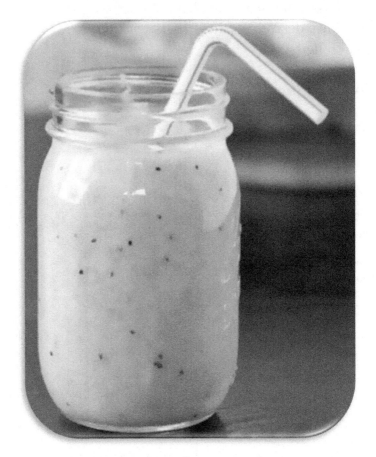

Preparation time: 10 minutes
Total time: 10 minutes
Servings: 1

Ingredients:

- 1 pear, chopped
- 1 kiwi, chopped
- 1 banana, sliced
- ½ cup coconut water

How to prepare:

1. Add all ingredients to a blender.
2. Blend until desired consistency is reached.
3. You can add more water if you want.
4. Serve chilled and enjoy!

Nutritional Values:

Calories 271
Total Fat 1 g
Saturated Fat 0 g
Cholesterol 0 mg
Sodium 131 mg
Total Carbs 69 g
Fiber 12 g
Sugar 41 g
Protein 4 g

Blueberry Banana Gooseberries Green Detox Smoothie

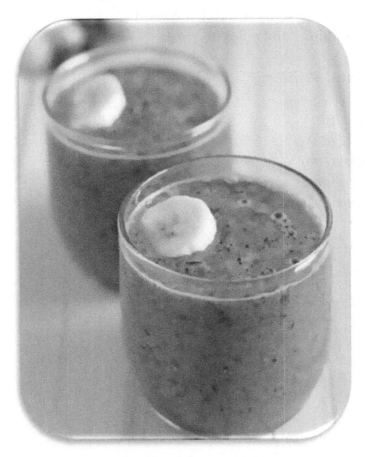

Preparation time: 10 minutes
Total time: 10 minutes
Servings: 2

Ingredients:

- 1½ cup almond milk
- 1 cup spinach
- 1 cup fresh blueberries

154

- 1 banana, sliced
- ½ cup cape gooseberries
- 1 tbsp flaxseed
- 1 tbsp almond butter

How to prepare:

1. Add all ingredients except all berries to a blender.
2. Blend for 30 seconds then add berries and blend until smooth.
3. Pour into serving glasses and serve.

Nutritional Values:
Calories 850
Total Fat 81.8 g
Saturated Fat 70.1 g
Cholesterol 0 mg
Sodium 57 mg
Total Carbs 33.7 g
Fiber 10.8 g
Sugar 18.5 g
Protein 9.7 g

Lemon Kale Detox Smoothie

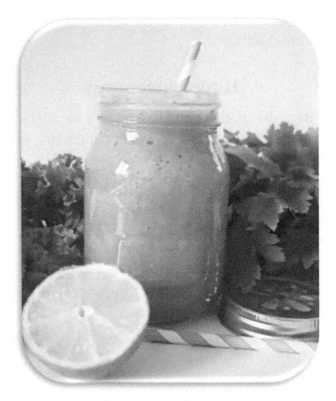

Preparation time: 10 minutes
Total time: 10 minutes
Servings: 2

Ingredients:

- 1 cup kale
- 1 cup parsley
- 1 cucumber, chopped
- 2 celery sticks
- 3 apples, chopped
- ½ lime, juiced
- 1 cup water

How to prepare:

1. Add all ingredients except lime juice to a blender.
2. Blend for 30 seconds.
3. Add in lime juice and blend for 30 seconds more.
4. Pour into serving glasses and enjoy.

Nutritional Values:
Calories 115
Total Fat 0.5 g
Saturated Fat 0.1 g
Cholesterol 0 mg
Sodium 36 mg
Total Carbs 29.1 g
Fiber 5.5 g
Sugar 19.1 g
Protein 2 g

Detoxifying Coconut Oil Smoothie

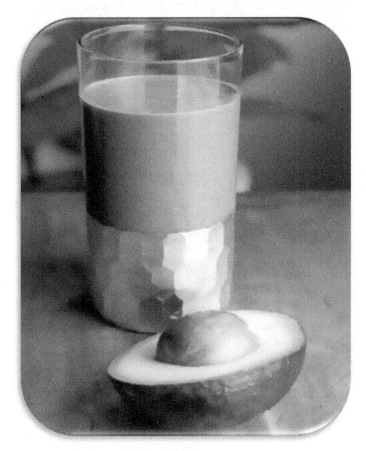

Preparation time: 10 minutes
Total time: 10 minutes
Servings: 2

Ingredients:

- 2 cups coconut milk
- 1 cup organic spinach, chopped
- 1 avocado, chopped
- 1 tbsp coconut oil

- 1 tsp spirulina powder
- 1 tsp lemon or lime juice
- 1 pinch sea salt

How to prepare:

1. Add all ingredients to a blender.
2. Blend for 30 seconds.
3. Pour into serving glasses and enjoy.

Nutritional Values:
Calories 828
Total Fat 83.8 g
Saturated Fat 60.8 g
Cholesterol 0 mg
Sodium 301 mg
Total Carbs 24.6 g
Fiber 12.5 g
Sugar 9 g
Protein 8.6 g
Potassium 1,244 mg

Monster Detox Smoothie

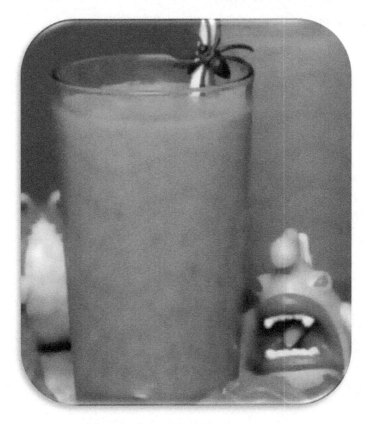

Preparation time: 10 minutes
Total time: 10 minutes
Servings: 2

Ingredients:

- 2 cups orange juice
- 1 cup raw spinach leaves
- 1 cucumber, chopped
- 1 apple, sliced
- 1 cup frozen banana, sliced

How to prepare:

1. Add all ingredients to a blender.
2. Blend until smooth.
3. Serve and enjoy.
4. You can add ice cubes if you want.

Nutritional Values:

Calories 251
Total Fat 0.9 g
Saturated Fat 0.2 g
Cholesterol 0 mg
Sodium 20 mg
Total Carbs 61.2 g
Fiber 6.3 g
Sugar 45.5 g
Protein 3.4 g

Broccoli Detox Smoothie

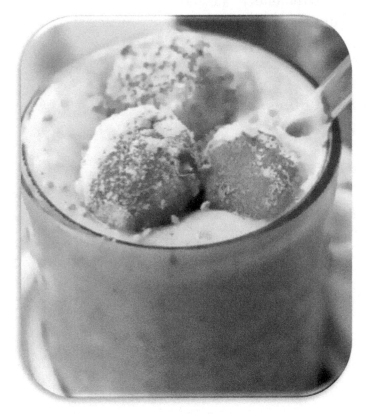

Preparation time: 10 minutes
Total time: 10 minutes
Servings: 1

Ingredients:

- ¾ cup broccoli florets, chopped
- 1 banana, sliced
- ½ cup pineapple, chunks
- ½ cup almond milk

How to prepare:

1. Add all ingredients to a blender.
2. Blend until desired consistency is reached.
3. Serve and enjoy.

Nutritional Values:

Calories 191
Total Fat 2 g
Saturated Fat 0 g
Cholesterol 0 mg
Sodium 187 mg
Total Carbs 43 g
Fiber 6 g
Sugar 24 g
Protein 4 g

Refreshing Green Detox Smoothie

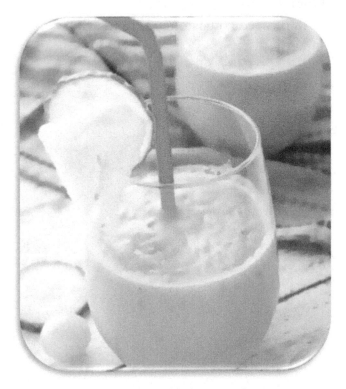

Preparation time: 10 minutes
Total time: 10 minutes
Servings: 1

Ingredients:

- 1 cup green grapes
- ½ cup cucumber, sliced
- ½ avocado, chopped
- 1 cup spinach
- 10 mint leaves
- ½ cup frozen pineapple
- 1 cup coconut water

How to prepare:

1. Add all ingredients to a blender.
2. Blend until desired consistency is reached.
3. Serve and enjoy.
4. You can add more coconut water if desired.

Nutritional Values:
Calories 397
Total Fat 21 g
Saturated Fat 4.5 g
Cholesterol 0 mg
Sodium 69 mg
Total Carbs 53 g
Fiber 16.5 g
Sugar 32.2 g
Protein 8 g

Vanilla Bean Green Detox Smoothie

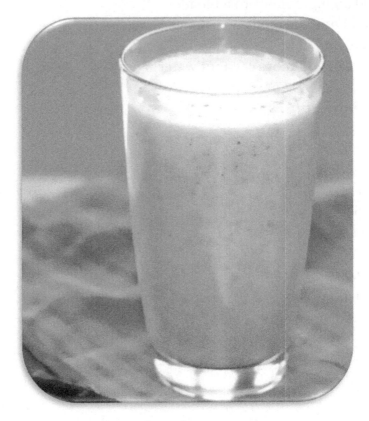

Preparation time: 10 minutes
Total time: 10 minutes
Servings: 1

Ingredients:

- 1 banana, frozen
- 1 cup shelled frozen edamame
- 2 tsp almond butter
- 1 vanilla bean
- 1 cup low-fat milk

How to prepare:

1. Add all ingredients to a blender.
2. Blend until desired consistency is reached.
3. Serve and enjoy.
4. You can add ice cubes if desired.

Nutritional Values:

Calories 480
Total Fat 16 g
Saturated Fat 4 g
Cholesterol 10 mg
Sodium 150 mg
Total Carbs 62 g
Fiber 11 g
Sugar 33 g
Protein 27 g

Morinaga Detoxifying Smoothie

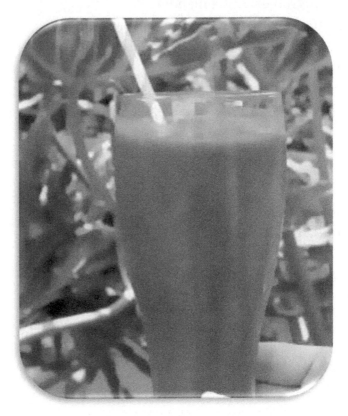

Preparation time: 10 minutes
Total time: 10 minutes
Servings: 2

Ingredients:

- 1 cup spinach
- 1 whole cucumber, chopped
- 1 lime, juiced
- 1 whole green apple, sliced
- 1 whole kiwi, sliced
- 1 tbsp moringa powder

How to prepare:

1. Add all ingredients to a blender.
2. Blend until desired consistency is reached.
3. Serve and enjoy

Nutritional Values:
Calories 129
Total Fat 5.6 g
Saturated Fat 0.8 g
Cholesterol 0 mg
Sodium 82 mg
Total Carbs 18.3 g
Fiber 2.9 g
Sugar 12.7 g
Protein 1.5 g

Green Detoxifying Pinacolato Smoothie

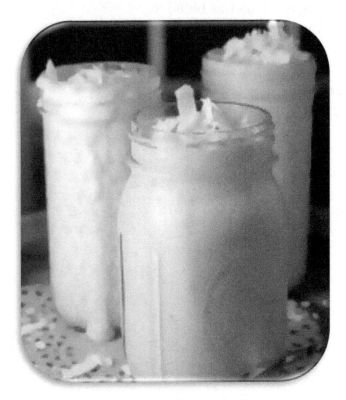

Preparation time: 10 minutes
Total time: 10 minutes
Servings: 2

Ingredients:

- 1 cup frozen banana
- ½ cup frozen pineapple
- ½ cup frozen mango
- 1 cup coconut milk
- 1 cup baby spinach
- 1 lime, juiced
- 2 tbsp toasted coconut for garnish

How to prepare:

1. Add all ingredients to a blender.
2. Blend until desired consistency is reached.
3. Serve and enjoy.

Nutritional Values:
Calories 512
Total Fat 31.3 g
Saturated Fat 26.8 g
Cholesterol 8 mg
Sodium 96 mg
Total Carbs 56.7 g
Fiber 5.1 g
Sugar 46.4 g
Protein 5.9 g

Alkaline Green Detox Smoothie

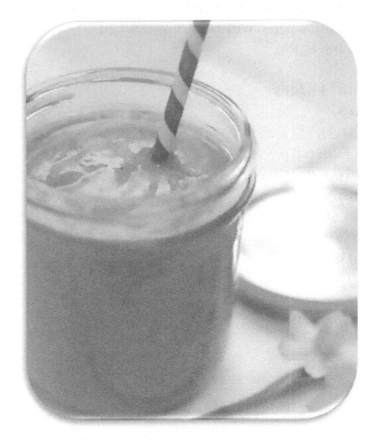

Preparation time: 10 minutes
Total time: 10 minutes
Servings: 1

Ingredients:

- 1 cucumber, chopped
- 3 medium kale leaves, torn
- 5 stems fresh mint
- 3 stems fresh parsley
- 1 piece fresh ginger

- 1 avocado
- 1 cup coconut water
- 1 lime, juiced
- 2 tsp Udo's oil
- 2 tbsp hemp seeds
- 3 drops stevia

How to prepare:

1. Add all ingredients to a blender.
2. Now blend the mixture until smooth.
3. Pour into serving glasses and enjoy.

Nutritional Values:
Calories 515
Total Fat 40.6 g
Saturated Fat 34.1 g
Cholesterol 0 mg
Sodium 89 mg
Total Carbs 37.3 g
Fiber 9.9 g
Sugar 17.3 g
Protein 8.4 g

Mango Turmeric Green Detox Smoothie

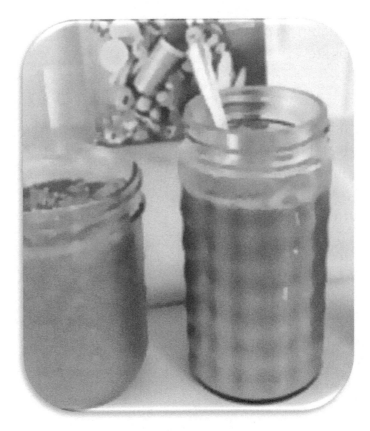

Preparation time: 10 minutes
Total time: 10 minutes
Servings: 1

Ingredients:

- 1 banana, chopped
- 1 cup almond milk
- 1 mango, chopped
- 2 tbsp fresh lemon juice

- 2 cups spinach
- 1 tbsp organic turmeric powder
- 1 inch piece ginger root

How to prepare:

1. Add all ingredients to a blender.
2. Now blend the mixture until smooth.
3. Pour into serving glasses and enjoy.

Nutritional Values:

Calories 909
Total Fat 60 g
Saturated Fat 51.7 g
Cholesterol 0 mg
Sodium 97 mg
Total Carbs 98.8 g
Fiber 16.6 g
Sugar 69.5 g
Protein 12 g

Green Tea Antioxidant Detox Smoothie

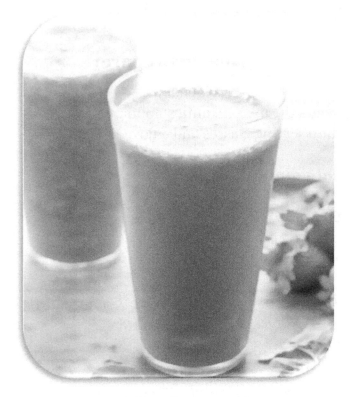

Preparation time: 10 minutes
Total time: 10 minutes
Servings: 2

Ingredients:

- 1 cup unsweetened almond milk
- ½ banana, peeled
- 1 cup spinach
- 1 cup strawberries, chopped
- ¾ cup ice
- 1 tbsp vanilla powder
- ½ tsp Matcha powder

How to prepare:

1. Add all ingredients to a blender.
2. Now blend the mixture until smooth.
3. Pour into serving glasses and enjoy.

Nutritional Values:

Calories 200
Total Fat 1 g
Saturated Fat 0 g
Cholesterol 0 mg
Sodium 0 mg
Total Carbs 29 g
Fiber 6 g
Sugar 16 g
Protein 14 g

Low Glycemic Detox Green Smoothie

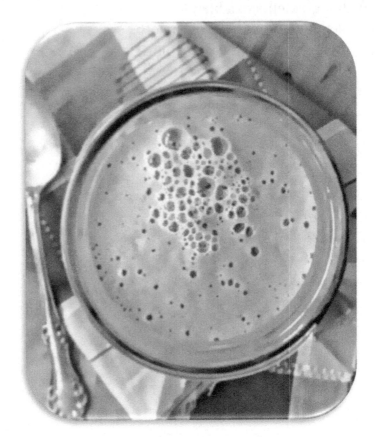

Preparation time: 10 minutes
Total time: 10 minutes
Servings: 2

Ingredients:

- 1 cucumber, chopped
- 5 ice cubes
- ½ avocado, chopped
- 1 tbsp almond butter
- 1 tbsp hemp seeds

- 1 chunk ginger root
- 1 tsp ground cinnamon
- 1 cup spinach
- ⅔ cups water

How to prepare:

1. Add all ingredients to a blender.
2. Now blend the mixture until smooth.
3. Pour into serving glasses and enjoy.

Nutritional Values:
Calories 187
Total Fat 14.8 g
Saturated Fat 2.5 g
Cholesterol 0 mg
Sodium 24 mg
Total Carbs 13.4 g
Fiber 6 g
Sugar 3.3 g
Protein 4.4 g

Tahini Fig Green Detox Smoothie

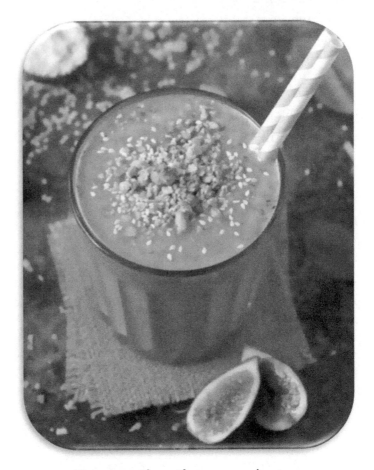

Preparation time: 10 minutes
Total time: 10 minutes
Servings: 1

Ingredients:

- 1 banana, chopped
- 2 figs, chopped
- 1 cup unsweetened almond milk
- ½ cup spinach

- 1 tbsp tahini
- 1 tbsp chia seeds
- 1 pinch cinnamon
- 5 large ice cubes

How to prepare:

1. Add all ingredients to a blender.
2. Now blend the mixture until smooth.
3. Pour into serving glasses and enjoy.

Nutritional Values:
Calories 471
Total Fat 21.1 g
Saturated Fat 2.6 g
Cholesterol 0 mg
Sodium 228 mg
Total Carbs 69.1 g
Fiber 19.4 g
Sugar 32.8 g
Protein 11.2 g

Chapter 5: Health Benefits of the of the 10-Day Green Smoothie Cleanse Weight Loss Diet Plan

This plan is known to be very beneficial in terms of health. Its main benefits are avoiding the following:

- Brain fog
- Indigestion
- Insomnia
- Allergies and sensitivities
- Bloating
- Poor digestion
- Low energy
- Constipation
- Fatigue
- Headaches
- Food cravings
- Infections
- Obesity
- Yeast infections
- Chronic pain

It is important to understand that this diet plan is not an alternative to any medical treatment. You cannot rule out the opinion or suggestions of a medical expert, doctor, nutritionist, etc. if you have any of the above mentioned health complications. These complications can be avoided befittingly by following the 10-Day cleanse but they cannot be TREATED with this diet plan. Always seek the opinion and advice of your doctor in case you suffer from any of those issues and do what they say first or at least discuss this plan with them to see if they approve of you trying it.

Conclusion

The 10-Day Green Smoothie Cleanse Weight Loss Diet Plan is known to have loads of medical benefits. The main goal is to detoxify your body to remove all toxins from your fat cells. Removing these toxins makes weight loss easier. The plan isn't hard to follow at all; you just need willpower to do it. If you can't follow the full cleanse variation of the 10-Day Cleansing Weight Loss Diet Plan, try the modified cleanse. Either way this cleanse is effective and beneficial.

Made in United States
North Haven, CT
02 February 2022

15552532R00104